Health Psychology
in Nursing Practice

SAGE was founded in 1965 by Sara Miller McCune to support the dissemination of usable knowledge by publishing innovative and high-quality research and teaching content. Today, we publish over 900 journals, including those of more than 400 learned societies, more than 800 new books per year, and a growing range of library products including archives, data, case studies, reports, and video. SAGE remains majority-owned by our founder, and after Sara's lifetime will become owned by a charitable trust that secures our continued independence.

Los Angeles | London | New Delhi | Singapore | Washington DC | Melbourne

Health Psychology
in Nursing Practice

Elizabeth Barley

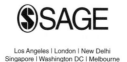

Los Angeles | London | New Delhi
Singapore | Washington DC | Melbourne

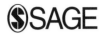

Los Angeles | London | New Delhi
Singapore | Washington DC | Melbourne

SAGE Publications Ltd
1 Oliver's Yard
55 City Road
London EC1Y 1SP

SAGE Publications Inc.
2455 Teller Road
Thousand Oaks, California 91320

SAGE Publications India Pvt Ltd
B 1/I 1 Mohan Cooperative Industrial Area
Mathura Road
New Delhi 110 044

SAGE Publications Asia-Pacific Pte Ltd
3 Church Street
#10-04 Samsung Hub
Singapore 049483

Editor: Becky Taylor
Editorial assistant: Charlène Burin
Production editor: Katie Forsythe
Copyeditor: Clare Weaver
Indexer: Silvia Benvenuto
Marketing manager: Camille Richmond
Cover design: Wendy Scott
Typeset by: C&M Digitals (P) Ltd, Chennai, India
Printed and bound by CPI Group (UK) Ltd,
Croydon, CR0 4YY

Library of Congress Control Number: 2015950696

British Library Cataloguing in Publication data

A catalogue record for this book is available from
the British Library

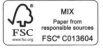

MIX
Paper from
responsible sources
FSC® C013604

ISBN 978-1-4739-1366-0
ISBN 978-1-4739-1367-7 (pbk)

At SAGE we take sustainability seriously. Most of our products are printed in the UK using FSC papers and boards.
When we print overseas we ensure sustainable papers are used as measured by the PREPS grading system.
We undertake an annual audit to monitor our sustainability.

CONTENTS

ABOUT THE AUTHOR

Elizabeth Barley (PhD CPsychol AFBPsS RGN) is an adult nurse, health psychologist and practitioner psychologist chartered by the British Psychological Society where she has associate fellow status. Elizabeth has been a registered general nurse since 1990. She was a staff nurse on a gynaecology ward before leaving to undertake a psychology degree. She funded her degree by working as an agency nurse. Through this, she gained experience on a range of medical and surgical wards, in occupational health and in the community.

Elizabeth completed her PhD at St George's, University of London when she studied the quality of life of adults with asthma. This involved collecting and analysing questionnaire data and conducting a judgement analysis study to determine which of the factors that affect quality of life are most important to patients. This and related research work and clinical practice enabled her to qualify as a health psychologist (under the 'grandparenting route').

Following completion of her PhD, Elizabeth moved to the Institute of Psychiatry (now the Institute of Psychiatry, Psychology and Neuroscience) at King's College London where she ran a clinical question-answering service which identified and appraised evidence in response to questions from a range of clinicians, including nurses. Whilst her two children were small, Elizabeth worked part-time as a research assistant and gained experience of qualitative and quantitative research methods and of systematic reviewing. During this time Elizabeth developed her interest in the mind–body interface and especially in how nurses can use health psychology to improve care for people with co-morbidities. She has numerous publications in this area and has presented her work to multidisciplinary audiences both nationally and internationally.

In 2012, Elizabeth joined the Florence Nightingale Faculty of Nursing and Midwifery at King's College London as a senior lecturer. Here she continued her research and indulged her love of teaching on a range of undergraduate and postgraduate (PGDip, MSc, Doctorate in Healthcare) courses as well as in supervising PhD students. Throughout her career, Elizabeth has undertaken health psychology-related clinical training and has maintained her clinical experience, for instance through delivering an intervention to patients with coronary heart disease as part of a randomised controlled trial and as an honorary therapist with an improving Access to Psychological Therapies service. Elizabeth is a visiting senior lecturer at the Florence Nightingale Faculty of Nursing and Midwifery, King's College London.

PUBLISHER'S ACKNOWLEDGEMENTS

The author and publisher would like to thank the following for their kind permission to republish material.

Figure 1.1: The Biomedical Model is adapted from a figure produced by Paul Leimkuehler and reproduced with kind permission of the American Academy of Orthotists and Prosthetists.

Figure 1.2: The Biophychosocial Model: a holistic model is an adaptation reproduced with kind permission of the American Academy of Orthotists and Prosthetists.

Figure 2.1: Adapted with permission of the copyright holder. Copyright 1986 Christine Padesky, www.MindOverMood.com

Table 2.1: Adapted by permission of the publisher from: Fishkind, A. (2002) Calming agitation with words, not drugs: 10 commandments for safety. *Current Psychiatry*. 1(4):32–34,37–39. Copyright © 2002 Frontline Medical Communications.

Table 2.2: Adapted from National Institute for Health and Care Excellence (2011) CG 123 Common mental health disorders: Identification and pathways to care. Manchester: NICE. Available from www.nice.org.uk/CG123. Reproduced with permission.

Figure 3.1: Reprinted from Clatworthy, J., Bowskill,R., Parham,R., Rank, T., Scott, J. and Horne, R. (2009) Understanding medication non-adherence in bipolar disorders using a Necessity-Concerns Framework. *Journal of Affective Disorders*. 116 (1–2): 51–5, with permission from Elsevier.

Table 3.1: Reprinted from Abdel-Tawab, R., James, D.H., Fichtinger, A., Clatworthy, J., Horne, R. and Davies, G. (2011) Development and validation of the Medication-Related Consultation Framework (MRCF). *Patient Education and Counseling*. 83(3): 451–7, Copyright 2011, with permission from Elsevier.

Figure 4.2: Published in Hall, P.A. and Fong G.T. (2007) Temporal self-regulation theory: A model for individual health behavior. *Health Psychology Review*. 1: 6–52. DOI: 10.1080/17437190701492437. Reprinted by permission of Taylor and Francis Ltd.

Box 7.1: The EAST Framework – four simple ways to apply behavioural insights reproduced with permission of The Behavioural Insights Team.

PREFACE

Our choice of a career in healthcare reflects our commitment to make the world a better place. We want to improve the lives of our patients and clients. As nurses, midwives, health visitors and allied health professionals our work is to support people to cope with illness, to prevent disease and, generally, to help people to be as well as they can be. This is true whatever the field or setting in which we work.

To ensure that we provide the best quality care, we have long since embraced the concept of evidence-based practice. Research evidence combined with our clinical expertise and our understanding of patient preferences ensures that the care and health advice we give is effective. However, even when people have an evidence-based treatment plan, they do not always follow it. Do all our patients take their prescribed medications as they should? Do they turn up for all their appointments or follow our diet, exercise or symptom management advice? In spite of a plethora of health education interventions, do we all eat healthily, drink only moderate amounts of alcohol, exercise enough, avoid tobacco and take up available preventative healthcare such as cancer screening? That, worldwide, the rates of preventable disability, morbidity and mortality are increasing provides the answer to these questions!

No single profession can address this alone. **Health psychology** is a discipline which has arisen to try to understand our health-related behaviour and to determine what support people need to be as well as they can be. In writing this book, I aim to illustrate how health psychology knowledge and techniques can complement the specialist skills and knowledge of nurses, midwives, health visitors and allied health professionals to help them to deliver the best possible care.

SCOPE OF THIS BOOK

This book is meant to introduce you to the discipline of health psychology. There are many health psychology textbooks available which cover a wide range of topics. As both a nurse and a health psychologist, I have given much consideration to which topics would be most useful to non-psychologist professionals. I decided to focus on those which have been identified through research and policy as challenges for nurses, midwives and health visitors and for anyone wanting to improve the health and **wellbeing** of patients and the public. There are therefore chapters on how health psychology relates to nursing, midwifery and health visiting practice in the context of: emotions and health (Chapter 2); improving self-management (Chapter 3); promoting healthy choices (Chapter 4); and managing enduring physical symptoms (Chapter 5). I also include a chapter on looking after yourself (Chapter 6), because we too deserve good health and wellbeing and without it, how can we care for others?

HEALTH PSYCHOLOGY AND HOW IT CAN HELP US AS NURSES, MIDWIVES OR HEALTH VISITORS

Psychology is the scientific study of people, the mind and behaviour. Health psychology is the application of psychological knowledge to the study of people's experience of health and illness. Health psychology research typically tries to predict or change how people will behave when they have a given illness, with the aim of improving physical and mental health outcomes and general **wellbeing**. These aims are shared by nurses, midwives and health visitors for their patients or clients.

Nurses, midwives and health visitors, of course, also conduct research. Combining what we know from nursing and health psychology enhances this research. This is especially the case in the field of behaviour change, which is important in the management of long-term conditions and health promotion – key areas of practice and research for many nurses, midwives and health visitors.

Specialist health psychologists may be part of the clinical team. Their role is to help people with the psychological and emotional aspects of illness or treatments and to support people with long-term conditions. This links closely with what nurses, midwives and health visitors do. At times we may need to provide very basic care, but a key part of our role is to ensure that patients or clients can self-manage in order to increase their independence, quality of life and their ability to cope in future. Health psychology theories and research, which predict how people may respond to illness and explain what is needed for people to manage their health, can help nurses, midwives and health visitors to do this.

THEORIES OF HEALTH AND BEHAVIOUR

To help you judge their value, as you read about theories of health and behaviour, bear in mind the information in Box 1.1 which summarises the properties of a good theory in social science.

Box 1.1: What makes a good theory in social science?

- Parsimony – explains a phenomenon in few terms as simply as possible
- Breadth – can be applied to a range of situations
- Accuracy – can produce testable predictions
- Falsifiable – it can be disproved
- Known **moderators** – specifies variables that tell you when relationships can and can't be expected
- Known **mediators** – specifies variables that tell you how or why a relationship occurs
- Fruitfulness – leads to new ideas

Most nurses, midwives and health visitors will be familiar with the biomedical and the biopsychosocial models of health.

The Biomedical Model

This **model**, or way of thinking about health, was dominant through most of the 20th century. It is a linear, unidirectional model where health is considered simply to be the absence of disease. Illness is seen as within the body, causing bodily symptoms that lead on to disability and restrictions on social life (Figure 1.1). The body can therefore be mended like a machine: removing part of a body or adding chemicals to it will lead to cure or avoidance of death.

However, the model was soon recognised as too simplistic and an alternative model – the biopsychosocial model – was proposed by psychiatrist George Engel (Engel, 1977) who advocated its use in research, teaching, and the provision of healthcare.

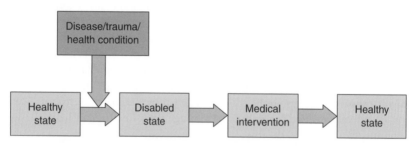

Figure 1.1   The Biomedical Model

Adapted from a figure produced by Paul Leimkuehler for the American Academy of Orthotists and Prosthetists.

The Biopsychosocial Model

This model recognises the contribution of biomedical, psychological and social factors to health (Figure 1.2). Biomedical factors include our genes, anatomy, physiology, bacteria and viruses; psychological factors may be our personality, behaviours and beliefs; social factors include social class, gender, ethnicity and socio-economic status.

How the Biopsychosocial Model Improves on the Biomedical Model

The biomedical model predicts an external cause of disease, but none may be found. For instance, in 'medically unexplained syndromes' such as irritable bowel syndrome, **chronic fatigue syndrome, fibromyalgia** and chronic low back pain, a person may experience very real and disabling symptoms but no medical reason can be identified. A biological cause for many severe mental illnesses has yet to be found.

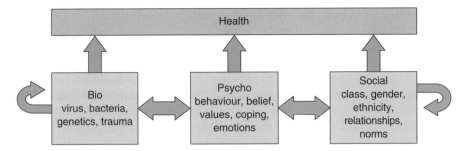

Figure 1.2 The Biopsychosocial Model: a holistic model

Adapted and reproduced with kind permission of the American Academy of Orthotists and Prosthetists.

The biopsychosocial model does not focus solely on cause, but recognises that beliefs and behaviours around illness can influence symptoms. We will look at this in more detail when we consider specific psychological theories.

The biomedical model also cannot explain individual variation in illness experience. For instance, two people with the same disease severity may report wide variation in their quality of life. The biopsychosocial model would predict that variation in psychological factors such as personality or **cognition**, or in social factors, such as available resources, are important. Compared to the other, one of the individuals may be more 'resilient' or able to distract themselves from symptoms, or they may have more family or practical support (someone to do the shopping) so that symptoms have less impact.

The 'placebo effect', where simply the expectation of cure can be beneficial, would fit with the biopsychosocial model which considers the impact of psychological factors on health (even if it does not explain them), but not the biomedical model, since no simple cause and effect process can be demonstrated.

The Biopsychopharmacosocial Model

Recently, a biopsychopharmacosocial model has been proposed (Clark and Clarke, 2014). This model builds on the biopsychosocial model to take into account how pharmaco-therapy can impact upon all aspects of patients' lives due to, for instance, side effects, beliefs around medications (the patients' and those of others) and the behaviours needed to adhere to a medication regimen. This model may be particularly relevant to those taking long-term daily medications such as people with mental illness or long-term conditions.

BEHAVIOUR CHANGE THEORIES IN HEALTH

The biopsychosocial model is therefore a general theory of how biomedical, psychological and social factors interact within health. Health psychology theories build on the biopsychosocial model by trying to predict or explain in more detail how specific biomedical, psychological and social factors interact to influence health or illness behaviours and outcomes. Theories differ in terms of their emphasis on cognitions (beliefs), affect (emotions or feelings) or habits, or on change processes or maintenance of ongoing behaviours.

Health psychologist Susan Michie and colleagues (2014) have identified no less than 83 theories concerned with behaviour change and considered useful when developing interventions to change behaviour. Several of the included theories, such as the 'Ecological Model for Preventing Type 2 Diabetes in Minority Youth' (Burnet et al., 2002) and the 'General Theory of Deviant Behaviour' (Kaplan et al., 1982), focus on very specific conditions, populations or behaviours. It is probably more helpful here to focus on broader health psychology theories, which, as nurses, midwives or health visitors, we can apply to a range of conditions and associated health behaviours.

The three models discussed focus on changing individual behaviour; theories of societal behaviour change will be considered briefly in Chapter 4 in relation to governments' or companies' attempts to change population or group behaviour.

The Health Belief Model (Rosenstock, 1966; Becker, 1974)

The Health Belief Model (HBM) predicts that people make decisions about their behaviour based on a rational weighing up of perceived pros and cons or 'costs and benefits analysis'. It is a 'cognitive model', which means that the role of beliefs is emphasised.

The HBM specifies the beliefs which predict how likely it is that someone will change their behaviour. These beliefs are:

- Perceived vulnerability – how 'at risk' a person feels
- Disease severity – how severe/unpleasant the person perceives a disease to be
- The costs of changing a behaviour – e.g. 'I will feel stressed if I stop smoking'
- The benefits of changing a behaviour – e.g. 'I will be able to wear my nice dress if I lose weight'
- Cues to action – triggers or prompts to change behaviour, either internal e.g. symptoms or external e.g. health advice from a nurse

Later developments of the HBM consider the influence of **'self-efficacy'** (the person's belief that they can change) and 'health **motivation**' (readiness to change). These factors involve the beliefs and influence of others so the HBM can now be termed a 'social cognition model' (see Box 1.2).

HBM Critical Appraisal and Evidence Base

The HBM predicts that if someone perceives a negative health outcome to be severe, sees themselves to be susceptible to it, considers the benefits of behaviours that reduce the likelihood of that outcome to be high, and perceives the barriers to adopting those behaviours to be low, then they will be likely to change their behaviour. If the model is correct, research evidence will show that these beliefs will predict actual behaviour.

In a systematic review, Carpenter (2010) found 18 studies, published between 1982 and 2007, which tested this in relation to treatment or health prevention behaviours. Carpenter focused on prospective longitudinal studies as an earlier similar review by

Harrison and colleagues (1992) suggested that retrospective studies may be biased since they tended to show significantly larger effect sizes than prospective studies. Carpenter's review found that beliefs around severity, benefits and barriers did predict the likelihood of future behaviour. Benefits and barriers were the strongest predictors; perceived susceptibility was a poor predictor. There were differences in effect for treatment versus health prevention behaviours and the length of time between measurement of beliefs and performance of behaviour appeared to moderate the effects. Carpenter proposes that more work is needed to identify the mediators and moderators between health beliefs and behaviour.

To determine whether the HBM is useful in healthcare practice we need to examine RCTs testing interventions informed by the model. Jones and colleagues (2014) identified 18 studies (16 RCTs; two before and after controlled trials, search conducted 2012), which tested the effect of HBM interventions on adherence to a range of health behaviours such as taking medications, following diets and making lifestyle changes. The quality of the included studies was rated by the authors as varying from high to low, although most of the studies did not report sufficient information for the authors to assess fully the risk of bias. The reviewers found that the majority of the studies (15/18) reported statistically significant improvements in adherence compared to control interventions.

Only six of the studies used all elements of the HBM. The interventions in the included studies mostly targeted beliefs around benefits, susceptibility and barriers. In contrast to Carpenter's review (2010), Jones and colleagues (2014) found no difference in effectiveness between interventions based on different beliefs. Carpenter's review included trials of any health behaviour whereas Jones et al.'s (2014) review only included interventions which addressed adherence to treatment; it is possible that the HBM, or elements of it, is better at predicting some kinds of behaviours than others. In addition, since few trials tested the full HBM it is possible that intervention success may be due to factors independent of the model, such as specific behaviour change techniques.

Evidence for the effectiveness of interventions informed by the HBM is therefore weak. However, there is evidence that the beliefs within the model can predict behaviour. As nurses, midwives and health visitors it will be useful for us to use this information to help understand why a particular patient may be finding it hard to make healthy choices. The importance of health beliefs is illustrated in the case example which relates health beliefs to the decision to take up breast cancer screening.

Case Example: Health beliefs and uptake of breast cancer screening

Jean is 50 years old and has been invited to attend for a mammography for the first time as part of a national breast cancer screening programme.

Jean's 'perceived vulnerability' is low; she thinks 'no one in my family has had this disease'. Her perception of 'disease severity' is high; she remembers 'my friend Vivien had breast cancer, chemotherapy was really horrible and the cancer could come back any time'.

(Continued)

(Continued)

Jean considers what would be involved if she accepted the invitation (her perceived costs); she thinks 'the procedure may be painful and I will have to take time off work'. She wonders if it is worth going for the mammogram (her perceived benefits); she thinks 'at least, if I do have breast cancer, it would be caught early and I may not have to have chemotherapy'.

After reading the leaflet that came with the invitation more fully and after talking to a colleague who has recently attended (cues to action), Jean decides she will go for her mammography.

Whether she actually attends may depend on how confident she is that she can organise time off work to have the procedure (self-efficacy).

Theory of Planned Behaviour (Ajzen, 1985, 1991; Ajzen and Madden, 1986) and Reasoned Action (Fishbein and Ajzen, 1975)

The Theory of Planned Behaviour (TPB) is a general theory of behaviour which has been very widely applied to health. It is a 'social cognition model' (see Box 1.2), so **attitudes** and beliefs of the individual and others are at its centre. It considers both change processes and maintenance behaviours.

It is developed from the Theory of Reasoned Action (TRA). Central to TRA is that intention to act is the best predictor of behaviour. Intentions are developed following an individual's evaluation of a behaviour and its expected outcomes. Their evaluation is influenced by their '**subjective norms**'. Subjective norms are the social pressures perceived by an individual as a result of their beliefs about what they think others think they should do. How much they want to do what others want is important too; social pressure will be higher if it is perceived as coming from respected or loved others. Figure 1.3 applies the TPB to stopping smoking.

The TPB adds the construct of 'perceived behavioural control' to the model. Perceived behavioural control is considered important to both behavioural intention and actual behaviour; it relates to the ease or difficulty with which an individual thinks they will be able to carry out a behaviour. As such, it is very similar to the concept of self-efficacy described in Box 1.2. Perceived behavioural control is informed by 'internal control factors', such as perceived or known skills, abilities, feeling informed, and by 'external control factors', such as perceived or known obstacles, and opportunities. Perceived internal and external control factors are derived from past experience. Figure 1.3 illustrates the TPB with an example of someone, whom the model would predict, is in a good position to stop smoking. It is possible to see that if any of the stated beliefs and attitudes were less positive the likelihood of stopping smoking would be reduced.

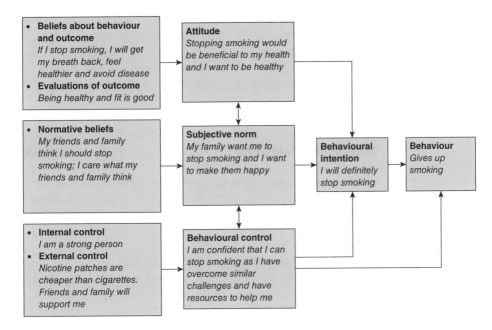

Figure 1.3 Theory of Planned Behaviour applied to stopping smoking (Ajzen, 1991)

TPB Critical Appraisal and Evidence Base

A systematic review by McEachan and colleagues (2011) identified 206 articles (search year 2010), including a range of study designs, which contained 237 independent empirical tests of the TPB. The strength of the review was that it included only prospective studies of all elements of the TPB in relation to a range of health or health risk behaviours. Various predictions of the model were supported: intention was the strongest predictor of prospective behaviour, demonstrating a medium to large effect; direct measures of attitudes and perceived behavioural control showed medium-sized relationships with behaviour; attitude was the strongest predictor of intention, followed by perceived behavioural control (direct) and then **social norms**; past behaviour showed medium to large correlations with behaviour and intention, and medium correlations with attitude and perceived behavioural control, and a small to medium relationship with social norms. Overall a meta-analysis indicated that the TPB explained 19.3 per cent of the variance in behaviour and 44.3 per cent of the variance in intention. This is a smaller number than an earlier slightly less rigorous meta-analysis found (Armitage and Conner, 2001), which had otherwise similar findings. These findings demonstrate that the TPB model is insufficient, as is any model, to fully explain behaviour change.

To address this McEachan and colleagues (2011) examined moderating factors and found that behaviour type moderated relationships among the model components, for instance, physical activity and dietary behaviours were best predicted by the model. The mean age of the sample was also important in relationships and in specific behaviours. Study methodology factors such as length of follow-up and type of outcome measure were also moderators, with larger effects found for shorter follow-up time periods and for outcomes measured by self-report compared with an objective measure.

Overall, there is some evidence for the ability of the TPB to predict behaviour, but the picture is complicated as other factors, not in the model, are also important. The strength of the TPB, compared with the HBM, is that, instead of assuming that people act in rational and coherent ways, an element of irrationality is included within the evaluations element, social and environmental factors are considered through the inclusion of social norms, and the importance of past behaviour is accounted for as part of perceived behavioural control.

There is much less evidence concerning the effectiveness of interventions informed by the TPB to change health behaviour, perhaps because guidance on developing concrete intervention strategies from the abstract theory is vague (French et al., 2013). Darker and colleagues (2010) developed an intervention to promote walking in the general public which was designed to alter perceived behavioural control and create walking plans. They tested whether the intervention increased TPB measures concerning walking more, planning and objectively measured walking in an RCT of 130 adults. They found that the intervention increased perceived behavioural control, attitudes, intentions and objectively measured walking from 20 to 32 minutes a day post intervention and at 6 weeks follow up. This was a well-designed study, but more experimental research is needed to test whether interventions informed by the TPB are effective for behaviours other than walking and in populations other than the general public. In the meantime, the model can be used to help us to consider systematically the myriad factors that make behaviour change in our patients more or less likely.

Box 1.2: Social cognition models

Based on Social Cognition Theory (Bandura, 1977, 1986).
  Behaviour is seen as governed by:

- Expectancies – situation outcome expectancy, behaviour may be dangerous; outcome expectancy, behaviour can reduce harm; self-efficacy expectancy, the person believes they can accomplish the desired behaviour
- Incentives – the consequences of the behaviour are important
- Social cognitions – beliefs about other people and the broader world

Stages of Change (Transtheoretical) Model: (Prochaska and DiClemente, 1983; Prochaska et al., 1992)

The Stages of Change Model (SCM) introduces the importance of 'readiness to change' to behaviour change models. It predicts that people at different stages of

vary slightly. Diagnosis requires at least one (DSM-5) or two (ICD-10) key symptoms (low mood, loss of interest and pleasure or loss of energy) to be present plus a number of other symptoms, such as significant weight loss or gain, physical agitation, fatigue or loss of energy, significant distress or impairment, feelings of worthlessness or excessive guilt, reduced concentration, indecisiveness. Symptoms should have been present for at least two weeks in sufficient severity for most of every day for a diagnosis to be made.

Point-prevalence (the proportion of a population experiencing the condition at the time of asking) and 12-month prevalence rates for depression of two to five per cent within the general population have been reported (Waraich et al., 2004). Lifetime prevalence (the likelihood of a condition occurring *ever* in a person's lifetime) has been found to be between seven per cent (Waraich et al., 2004) and 17 per cent (Kessler et al., 2005b). It is increasingly recognised that 'subthreshold' symptoms – symptoms of depression that do not reach the level necessary for diagnosis – are disabling and distressing if they persist (NICE CG90, 2009a). Subthreshold symptoms are more common than depression diagnoses.

ANXIETY – DEFINITION AND PREVALENCE

Anxiety is a commonly experienced emotion, but is not termed a disorder, unless symptoms are present for at least six months and cause clinically significant distress or impairment in social, occupational or other important areas of functioning (NICE CG113, 2011a). DSM-5 (American Psychiatric Association, 2013) lists a number of anxiety disorders which have excessive anxiety as the primary symptom and which have specific diagnostic criteria such as specific phobia, social anxiety disorder, panic disorder, agoraphobia, generalised anxiety disorder, substance/medication-induced anxiety disorder, anxiety disorder due to another medical condition, other specified anxiety disorder, unspecified anxiety disorder, separation anxiety disorder and selective mutism.

Generalised anxiety disorder is the most common anxiety disorder and is characterised by excessive worry associated with heightened tension (NICE CG113, 2011a). Anxiety disorders have been found in large-scale studies to have a lifetime prevalence of nearly 30 per cent (Kessler et al., 2005b). As with depression, subthreshold persistent anxiety symptoms such as irritability, restlessness, fatigue, muscle tension, poor concentration and problems sleeping are common and can be extremely debilitating.

COMMON MENTAL DISORDERS – DEFINITION AND PREVALENCE

Common mental disorder (CMD) is the term used to categorise those psychological problems which occur relatively frequently in populations. In contrast to the psychoses (serious mental illnesses such as schizophrenia and bipolar affective disorder), CMDs do not involve a loss of contact with reality, or major disturbances in thought processes, or an inability to recognise symptoms as abnormal or an illness.

CMDs include depression, generalised anxiety disorder, panic disorder, obsessive-compulsive disorder, post-traumatic stress disorder and social anxiety disorder (NICE GC123, 2011b). It is helpful to consider depression and anxiety under this umbrella term since their symptoms often co-exist and people frequently experience more than one of these conditions during their lifetime (Kessler, 2000; Kessler et al., 2005b). A diagnosis of 'mixed anxiety and depressive disorder' is the most commonly occurring CMD, with a point prevalence of nine per cent (McManus et al., 2009). It is characterised by anxiety and depressive symptoms, which are co-occurring and subthreshold.

CMDs are a major cause of suffering and disability for the people who experience them, as well as adversely affecting family and carers. People with these conditions have considerably increased health service costs (Katon et al., 2003). Lifetime prevalence estimates for CMDs suggest that around a quarter of people will experience one of these conditions at some point (Kessler et al., 2005a).

Predictors of Common Mental Disorders

Knowledge of the predictors of CMDs is useful for nurses, midwives and health visitors as it will alert us to patients who may be at increased risk of disorder. A large body of literature exists which details this: for England a comprehensive source of information is the Adult Psychiatric Morbidity Survey (McManus et al., 2009) of a representative sample of people aged 16 years and over living in private accommodation.

- Gender

Depression and all anxiety disorders are between one and a half and two and a half times as common in women as they are in men (Bebbington, 1998; Goodwin et al., 2005; McManus et al., 2009).

- Socioeconomic factors

As with many other health problems, mental health is worse in those with lower socioeconomic status; people in the lowest socioeconomic group are approximately twice as at risk as those in the highest group (McManus et al., 2009).

- Ethnicity

International studies provide inconsistent findings in relation to CMD prevalence and ethnicity (Bhugra and Mastrogianni, 2004; Asnaani et al., 2010). This inconsistency may be due to the effects of socioeconomic factors as well as to the methods used for disorder identification. In England, women of South Asian origin have been found to have higher rates of depression, panic and generalised anxiety disorder than other groups (McManus et al., 2009).

- Past history of CMD

A past history of anxiety or depression is a particularly important predictor of further episodes of these problems as relapse is common (Kessler et al., 2005b). The person's past history will also provide you with an indication of the kind of support and management strategies that are most likely to be acceptable and effective for them.

• Alcohol misuse

Alcohol misuse is commonly associated with mental health problems, especially with anxiety problems (Kessler et al., 2005a), so drinking habits should always be discussed when assessing patients.

• Antenatal and postnatal period

Women are more likely to experience depression and anxiety symptoms during the perinatal period, though there is little clear evidence that depression or anxiety disorder prevalence is higher during this period (Gavin et al., 2005; NICE, 2014b). However, since the potential consequences of maternal mental health problems are especially serious, healthcare professionals should be alert to potential problems throughout this period.

• Medical illness

Medical illness is an important risk factor for CMDs. People with long-term conditions (LTCs) have been found to have higher rates of depression and/or anxiety in a number of studies (Moussavi et al., 2007). People with LTCs who also have mental health problems tend to have worse physical outcomes, greater disability, and higher rates of death (Benton et al., 2007).

STRESS, ANGER AND GRIEF

Unlike depression and anxiety, stress, anger and grief are not usually associated with clinical diagnoses. They are normal emotional states, which are appropriate in many situations; as with depression and anxiety, they are only considered troublesome when they significantly impair functioning or when they influence health. We will consider the impact of stress, anger and grief on health in a later section, but first a brief overview of how psychologists view these emotions may be helpful.

Stress

We use the term 'stress' in many ways, for instance to describe feelings of being under pressure, overwhelmed by life demands or events or of tension. Stress is a complex construct and much literature is devoted to understanding it (see Further Reading); here we provide an overview. Early psychological theories conceptualise stress as a response to an external 'stressor' (a threat or new demand which feels challenging to the individual). Most people have heard of the 'fight or flight **model**' (Cannon, 1932) where, in response to threat, the body experiences increased arousal of the autonomic nervous system and release of adrenaline and endorphins which enable the individual to respond quickly, either by fleeing or attacking depending on the situation. Selye (1956) described the stress response in three stages, which he called the 'General Adaptation System'. Stage 1 is the 'alarm response' – the physiological arousal which prepares the individual for action; Stage 2 is 'resistance' – which is associated with coping and attempts to reduce the effects of alarm, corticosteroids continue to be released during this period to provide the body with energy and to stimulate its defence mechanisms; Stage 3 is 'exhaustion' – which happens after continual **exposure** to stressors and when the body cannot maintain resistance. This can happen suddenly, in extreme cases resulting in collapse or death, or slowly which results in stress-related illness, which we will consider later.

Life experiences have been defined by psychologists as stressors. The 'Schedule of Recent Experiences' (Holmes and Rahe, 1967) is an early example of a measure of stress which lists an extensive range of life changes or events such as 'death of a spouse', 'pregnancy', 'change in number of family get-togethers' – the number of experienced events was considered to indicate the level of stress. Later weightings, derived from research, were added to events to avoid the situation where someone who had experienced a very major event could score similarly to someone with a few more minor events. Problems with this approach are that it does not consider: 1) the individual's interpretation, for instance, one person may welcome pregnancy whereas another may not; 2) that stressors may interact with one another, for instance, moving house and getting married may be seen as two separate stressors (which added up increase overall stress), but the joy of moving house to live with a new spouse may cancel out the stress effects; 3) the duration of stressors, for instance, some life events are short lived whereas others, such as illness, may be **chronic**. Life events should therefore be considered in the context of the individual's ongoing stressors and social resources (e.g. **social support**, finances, etc.) (Moos and Swindle, 1990).

Such stimulus (stressor) and response (stress) models of stress, however, suggest that the individual passively reacts to stressors. This is clearly problematic as different people respond differently to the same event and find different things stressful which means that individual variation is important. This is addressed in the 'Transactional Model of Stress' (Lazarus, 1974; Lazarus and Folkman, 1984). In this model the role of the individual's appraisal is emphasised: 'primary appraisal' being the individual's judgement of the stressor, i.e. how threatening, challenging or dangerous it is; 'secondary appraisal' being the individual's judgement of their ability to cope with the stressor, i.e. can they alter, avoid or prevent the situation? This can be summarised:

Stress = perceived threat > perceived ability to cope.

⚙ Activity: Reflection

You will know from Chapter 1 that people's perceptions are influenced by numerous factors. Consider which factors may influence perceptions of threat and ability to cope. (Examples are given at the end of this chapter.)

However, this model assumes that the individual behaves rationally, whereas people under stress often behave irrationally, for instance, through the process of denial or through patterns of distorted thinking (see below and Box 2.1) which are common in distressed people. The concept of 'secondary gain', such as when stress is used as an excuse to miss work (whether this is a conscious or unconscious process), is also ignored. The key is to remember that many factors contribute to how stressed an individual feels and that different individuals will respond differently to the same stressor. Knowing this will help us as nurses, midwives and health visitors to provide person-centred care through avoidance of assumptions concerning what is 'appropriate' behaviour in a given situation.

Anger

The complexities of operationalising anger are well recognised by psychologists, though attempts at definition tend to include three related constructs: anger, hostility and aggression (Martin et al., 2000b). Anger is typically described as an 'affective' or emotional state varying from mild irritation to fury or rage; aggression is considered a behavioural expression of angry affect which may be verbal such as shouting or physical as in assault; hostility is viewed as a cognitive trait or negative **attitude** directed towards others. Despite important differences between these constructs, these terms often are used in research interchangeably and their inter-relationship remains poorly delineated (Martin et al., 2000b; Chida and Steptoe, 2009). Nevertheless, conceptualising the constructs in terms of 'ABC' (affect, behaviour, **cognition**) is useful to healthcare professionals who need to manage others' (or their own) anger since, if we can identify the most troublesome aspect, intervention can be targeted at feelings/affect (e.g. encouraging acceptance of the emotion, or acknowledging the validity of feelings), behaviour (e.g. walking away, restraint) or the beliefs causing anger (e.g. challenging unhelpful beliefs by providing information or other evidence).

Grief

As stated previously, grief is a normal emotion associated with loss, most severely perhaps with the death of a loved one, but also with loss of other things of value such as opportunity, youth, functional ability or health. The terms grief and bereavement are used inconsistently in research, but generally bereavement may be considered the fact of loss and grief the affective, behavioural and cognitive reaction to it; 'mourning' relates specifically to behavioural manifestations of grief which are influenced by social and cultural rituals (Zisook and Shear, 2009).

Stage models of grief have been proposed. The Kübler-Ross model (Kübler-Ross, 1969) which describes stages of denial, anger, bargaining, depression and acceptance is commonly cited, but its application to grief may be misplaced since this was originally conceptualised as a model of dying, i.e. the responses of terminally ill people to awareness of their own death. This may explain the lack of empirical support found for this model (National Cancer Institute, 2014). Some evidence has been found for a 5-stage model incorporating disbelief, yearning, anger, depression and acceptance (Maciejewski et al., 2007).

Stage models are appealing since an understanding of how individuals grieve may aid in determining whether someone's adjustment to loss is normal or not. However, it is now generally accepted that individual variation in normal grieving is immense and not everyone will progress through the same stages at the same rate, though several studies have found the intensity of grief to reduce considerably during the first six months (Shear et al., 2011). The **acute**, early phase of normal grief can be extremely painful and consuming and functioning may be disrupted, but normal grief is usually time limited and does not require formal treatment for it to become 'integrated' and for functioning to return to normal (Zisook and Shear, 2009). In fact, a 'review of reviews' suggests that 'there is now sufficient evidence to conclude that generic interventions, targeted toward the general population of the bereaved, are likely to be unnecessary and largely unproductive' (Jordan and Neimeyer, 2003).

There has been considerable debate concerning whether grief can ever be considered a disorder. Researchers have described a lack of transition from acute to integrated grief as 'prolonged' or 'complicated' grief (Prigerson et al., 2009; Shear et al., 2011). About seven per cent of bereaved older adults may develop complicated grief (Shear et al., 2011). DSM-5 has acknowledged this research and includes, in the chapter on 'Conditions for Further Study', a category of 'persistent complex bereavement-related disorder'. Diagnosis requires that, at 12 months post loss, there is present at least one out of four of 'separation distress' symptoms (yearning/longing, intense sorrow, preoccupation with the deceased, preoccupation with the death's circumstances), and at least six out of 12 additional symptoms including difficulty accepting, shocked/stunned/numb, difficulty positively reminiscing, bitterness/anger, self-blame, avoidance of reminders, difficulty trusting, wanting to join the deceased, loneliness/detachment, meaningless-ness/emptiness, role confusion or feeling part of oneself died, and difficulty pursuing interests or plans. These symptoms occur in normal grief, so 'it is the prolonged intensity rather than a trajectory of resolution that suggests pathology' (Wakefield, 2013: 172). A review of the literature on complicated grief (Shear et al., 2011) suggests that treatment that identifies complicated grief, addresses complications and facilitates the natural health process may be effective. The review also suggested that antidepressants may be helpful, particularly in combination with psychological therapy. However, this was not a fully systematic review; further trials of psychological therapy for complicated grief are ongoing and may or may not support these findings.

ASSOCIATIONS BETWEEN TROUBLESOME EMOTION AND HEALTH

CMDs, stress, anger and grief have all been found by research to be associated with ill health.

CMDs and health

People with long-term conditions such as coronary heart disease (CHD), diabetes, asthma, chronic obstructive pulmonary disease (COPD), renal disease, epilepsy, Parkinson's disease, HIV/AIDS and cancer have been found to have higher rates of depression and/or anxiety in a number of studies (Moussavi et al., 2007; Steptoe, 2007). People with a long-term condition who also have mental health problems also tend to have worse physical outcomes, greater disability, and higher rates of death (Benton et al., 2007). People who are depressed after a coronary event are twice as likely to have a further coronary event (odds ratio 2.0) and nearly three times more likely to die (odds ratio 2.6) than people who are not depressed (Barth et al., 2004; van Melle et al., 2004; Stafford et al., 2007).

Anger and Health

Despite the difficulties of operationalising anger for research purposes, there is a large body of research considering the impact of anger on health – most of this focuses on heart disease. Early research focused on anger as a personality trait and suggested that 'type A behaviour', which is characterised by hostility, intense ambition, competitive drive, constant preoccupation with deadlines and a sense of time urgency, was associated with heart disease. However, a comprehensive systematic review has indicated no real evidence for this association (Myrtek, 2001). Later research has focused more simply on anger or hostility. A well-conducted systematic review of prospective cohort studies, with a follow-up period of more than 1 year (Rutledge and Hogan, 2002), found moderate support for anger (and anxiety and depression), however it was measured, as a predictor of hypertension development. Review evidence also suggests that anger and hostility are associated with CHD outcomes both in healthy (evidence from 25 studies) and CHD populations (evidence from 19 studies) (Chida and Steptoe, 2009).

Evidence for the role of anger in causing other conditions is, however, sparse. Anger inhibition or suppression has been studied extensively in relation to pain and to cancer. However, early reports suggesting that 'trait anger-in' (self-reported tendency to inhibit anger expression) is associated with both acute and chronic pain severity have been questioned due to inadequate definition of the anger-in trait and overlap with measures of negative affect (Burns et al., 2008). Similarly, anger-in has been proposed as an antecedent of cancer (Thomas et al., 2000). A prospective cohort study over 9 years (n=19,730 adults) (White et al., 2007), suggested that anger control and negative affect were not associated with breast cancer, melanoma, or total cancer risk, but that they may have a small role in risk of prostate, colorectal and lung cancer, though further research is needed to confirm this.

Stress and Health

Stressful events such as terrorist attacks and earthquakes have been found to produce both profound and sustained increases in blood pressure (Parati et al., 2001; Vaccarino et al., 2007; Hamer et al., 2008). Unsurprisingly, prolonged stress such as socioeconomic adversity, social isolation and workplace stress are shown by review evidence to be implicated in CHD (Steptoe and Kivimaki, 2013).

Grief and Health

In a cohort study of 112 bereaved spouses (Ott, 2003), the authors classified 29 as having complicated grief (CG); those with CG were found to have worse overall mental health status over 18 months than those not classified this way but there was no significant difference in self-reported physical health symptoms between the groups. In a second study of 328 bereaved spouses (all women) (Utz et al., 2012), considerable **somatic** symptoms were reported shortly after bereavement, but no major health decline was observed over the following 18 months. Poor health at the time of bereavement appeared to be associated with higher risk of complicated grief and major depressive disorder. In bereaved parents, unresolved grief may to be linked to ill health: in a survey of 449 Swedish parents who had lost a child as a result of cancer 4 to 9 years earlier, those who reported not having worked through their grief reported significantly worse psychological health (fathers: RR, 3.6; 95 per cent CI, 2.0 to 6.4; mothers: RR, 2.9; 95 per cent CI, 1.9 to 4.4) and physical health (fathers: RR, 2.8; 95 per cent CI, 1.8 to 4.4; mothers: RR, 2.3; 95 per cent CI, 1.6 to 3.3) compared with those who reported having worked through their grief (Lannen et al., 2008). It appears that poor adjustment to grief, rather than grief *per se*, may be a risk factor for ill health, though more research is needed to confirm this.

Pathways between Troublesome Emotion and Health

Despite clear associations between troublesome emotion and ill health, the pathways between the two are not fully understood. Proposed biological pathways include higher cardiovascular stress reactivity, reduced heart rate variability, reduced heart rate recovery, dysfunctional hypothalamic-pituitary-adrenal axis, greater cortisol reactivity to stress, increased awakening and daytime cortisol levels, increased inflammatory mediators and increased platelet reactivity. However, in a prospective study of 6,576 healthy men and women (Hamer et al., 2008) the association between psychological distress and CVD risk was largely explained by behavioural processes (such as cigarette smoking, physical activity, alcohol intake), and pathophysiological factors accounted for only a modest amount of the variance. Further research concerning pathways in conditions other than heart disease is needed.

Whatever the direction of causality, there is compelling evidence that troublesome emotion is linked with ill health. This reinforces the importance of nurses, midwives and health visitors taking an holistic approach to care. A good understanding of troublesome emotions, how to screen for CMDs and how we can help patients to manage their emotions better will help.

UNDERSTANDING TROUBLESOME EMOTION

Cognitive Factors in Troublesome Emotion

Psychologists have long established that how we think, feel and react (behaviourally and physiologically) is linked. This is illustrated in the 'thoughts, feelings, behaviour and physiology cycle' shown in Figure 2.1.

In **health psychology**, the dominant model of emotional disorder is the cognitive model, which is based on a cognitive theory of **psychopathology** first described by psychologist Aaron Beck (Beck, 1967). The cognitive model describes how people's perceptions of and beliefs about situations influence their emotional, behavioural

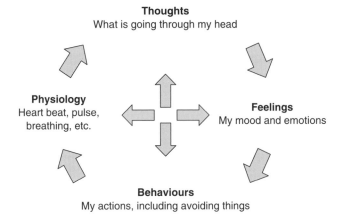

Figure 2.1 The thoughts, feelings, behaviour and physiology cycle

Figure adapted with permission of the copyright holder. Copyright 1986 Christine A. Padesky, www.MindOverMood.com

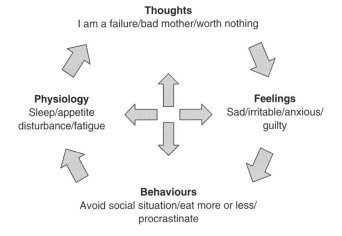

Figure 2.2 The thoughts, feelings, behaviour, physiology cycle applied to depression

and physiological reactions. When an individual is distressed, the model proposes that their perceptions and thoughts are distorted or dysfunctional and that by 'correcting' their thinking, so that it is more balanced and better reflects what is actually happening, their distress will improve. Figure 2.2 shows a thoughts, feelings, behaviour and physiology cycle for someone who is depressed.

The content of thoughts will depend on the individual's circumstance. Our minds are constantly forming opinions and interpreting events. Sometimes we may not be fully conscious of our thoughts and habitual ways of thinking can occur. If these habitual thinking patterns are overly negative or irrational we can become distressed. Common '**thinking errors**', or distorted ways of thinking, which contribute to troublesome emotion have been identified, see Box 2.1.

Box 2.1: Common thinking errors

All-or-nothing thinking:

If a situation isn't absolutely perfect – thinking of it as a complete failure.

Black-and-white thinking:

Thinking in extremes and neglecting the more likely middle ground.

Overgeneralising:

Drawing overall negative conclusions based on one incident.

Selective thinking:

Focusing on the negative and rejecting the positive; seeing only the bad in something or dwelling on negative events and ignoring the positive ones; explaining away positives or putting them down to luck.

Jumping to conclusions:

Making a judgement and assuming it is right with few facts to back it up.

Mind-reading:

Assuming you know what other people are thinking or guessing their opinion without actually asking them.

Predicting the future:

Assuming a negative outcome before an event has even occurred.

Catastrophising:

Seeing things as a complete disaster or totally impossible to cope with.

Should statements:

Having rules about how you or others 'should' behave and making judgements based on these rules, which leads to being overly critical.

Typical thinking errors and irrational beliefs have been associated with different troublesome emotions. In severe anxiety or panic, people commonly 'catastrophise' their bodily sensations (Clark, 1986). For instance, a stressful situation usually causes the heart to beat faster; instead of interpreting this as a normal reaction, an anxious or panicking person may believe that they are about to have a heart attack. This may lead them to avoid stressful situations (known as **avoidance behaviour**) or to carry out other behaviours designed to protect them against the thing they fear (known as **safety behaviours**) such as drinking alcohol to calm nerves or avoiding shaking hands for fear of germs. These avoidance and safety behaviours help people to feel better in the short term, but in the long term only maintain the irrational beliefs, unhelpful behaviours and troublesome emotions (as depicted in the 'thoughts, feelings, behaviour and physiology cycle').

⚙ **Activity: Reflection**

Try to identify thinking errors which may perpetuate different troublesome emotions. For example:

Anger: My husband/wife ALWAYS interrupts me (overgeneralising); the nurse SHOULD understand exactly how I feel (should statements).

Anxiety: If I don't get that job, my wife will leave me, I'll lose my home, I'll never be happy... (catastrophising/predicting the future).

Grief: Janet crossed the road when she saw me – I am so miserable to be with that she wants to avoid me (mind reading, jumping to conclusions – Janet may have been in a rush!).

Behavioural Factors in Troublesome Emotion

A large body of research identifies a range of behaviours that are associated with troublesome emotion, with most focusing on anxiety and depression. However, cause and effect relationships are unclear – that is we do not know whether these unhealthy behaviours are **depressogenic** or **anxiogenic** (see Box 2.2 for potential physiological pathways), or whether individuals genetically predisposed to depression or anxiety are more likely also to adopt these behaviours (Hamer et al., 2008). Nevertheless, there is evidence, in many cases, that if the individual stops the unhealthy behaviour, their mood improves.

Box 2.2: Potential physiological pathways between unhealthy behaviours and troublesome emotion

Tobacco smoking – is associated with neuroadaptations in nicotinic pathways in the brain which are associated with depressed mood, agitation and anxiety shortly after a cigarette is smoked (Benowitz, 2010).

Alcohol – Alcohol blocks the NMDA (N-methyl-D-aspartate) receptor, opposing glutamate, which causes amnesia and other depressant effects. Its effect on serotonin is linked to pleasurable effects, but differing brain serotonin levels may distinguish between anxious and aggressive alcohol users (McIntosh and Chick, 2004).

Inactivity – Physical activity improves mood by causing changes in endorphin and monoamine levels or by reducing levels of the stress hormone cortisol. It also stimulates the growth of nerve cells and the release of proteins, such as brain-derived

(Continued)

(Continued)

growth neurotrophic factor, which are known to improve the health and survival of nerve cells. Other physiological effects include: increased core temperature and cerebral blood flow, reduced muscular tension, and neurotransmitter efficiency (DH, 2004; Cooney et al., 2013).

Social support – has been linked to better immune functioning and to immune-mediated inflammatory processes (Holt-Lunstad et al., 2010); lack of social support may then be associated with systemic inflammation, which is in turn associated with depression (Berk et al., 2013).

Obesity – Obesity may disrupt the normal hormonal pathways causing increased hunger and food intake (Zametkin et al., 2004), but only 10 per cent of child obesity cases have been found to have been caused by systemic medical conditions, such as genetics or hormonal causes (National Obesity Observatory, 2011).

Cigarette smoking – Smokers commonly report smoking to improve their mood, help them to relax and to relieve stress (McEwen et al., 2008; Fidler and West 2009). However, smoking is strongly associated with diagnosis of mental disorder, particularly in heavy smokers and those who are more dependent (Coulthard et al., 2002; Royal College of Physicians, 2013). Smoking is also associated with self-reported psychological distress in healthy populations (Hamer et al., 2008).

A health belief that smoking is beneficial to mood helps perpetuate smoking behaviour (West et al., 2001; Ferguson et al., 2005), especially since smoking can reduce feelings of irritability in the short term (Parrott, 1999). Healthcare professionals who share this health belief may be reluctant to advise patients under stress or who are experiencing mental health problems to stop smoking. However, a well-conducted systematic review (Taylor et al., 2014) of studies (n=26) assessing mental health before stopping smoking and at least six weeks post cessation or baseline showed that stopping smoking is associated with reduced depression, anxiety, stress, improved mood and quality of life compared with continuing to smoke. This was true in people with and without a mental health diagnosis.

Alcohol – Heavy or binge drinking can be a mechanism for coping with stress or anxiety, including in young people (Newbury-Birch et al., 2009). However, alcohol has a depressant effect and can cause people to be aggressive (see Box 2.2), so drinking only makes matters worse. Excessive drinking is strongly associated with major depression (Sullivan et al., 2005).

Physical inactivity – Physical inactivity is a predictor of psychological distress (Hamer et al., 2008; Smith and Blumenthal 2013). Physical activity may influence mood through both physiological (see Box 2.2) and psychological pathways. Psychological pathways proposed (DH, 2004; Cooney et al., 2013) include improvements in perceptions of competence or confidence about the body and its capabilities; increased self-esteem, sense of achievement or self-efficacy; enhanced mastery and self-determination; diversion from negative thoughts and social contact during exercise.

A Cochrane review (Cooney et al., 2013) of 39 studies of exercise for depression found that exercise was moderately more effective than no treatment for improving depressive symptoms and similarly as effective as pharmacological or psychological therapy, though more evidence is needed to confirm this.

Over eating/Obesity – An overview of evidence on the relationship between obesity and mental health for adults and children in the UK was published by the National Obesity Observatory in 2011. They report findings that obese persons had a 55 per cent increased risk of developing depression and that depressed persons had a 58 per cent increased risk of becoming obese; a weak but positive association between obesity and anxiety disorders was also found. The evidence was strong in adults and teenagers; there was also weak evidence to support the association between obesity and poor mental health in younger children.

The findings of the report (National Obesity Observatory, 2011) suggest a bi-directional association between mental health problems and obesity, with mediating factors including: low self-esteem, stigma, dieting and weight cycling, medication and hormonal and functional impairment. Factors associated with mental health problems which may lead to obesity included: unhealthy lifestyles, medication and lack of social support.

Socialising/Social Support – Human beings are social animals. A potential physiological pathway between social support and mood is shown in Box 2.2. Psychological models have also been proposed (Cohen et al., 2000). The 'buffering hypothesis' suggests that social relationships provide resources, such as information, emotional support and tangible help that promote healthy responses to life stressors such as illness or life events. The benefits of social support therefore moderate the negative effects of stressors. The 'main effects model' suggests a more direct effect of social support, proposing that it facilitates healthier behaviours such as exercise, healthy eating, not smoking and treatment adherence, for instance, through modelling or **social norms**. Social support may also increase self-esteem and provide purpose, which are associated with improved mood.

The association of social support with depression has been studied particularly in older people, with a systematic review of 37 studies (Schwarzbach et al., 2014) concluding that qualitative aspects of social support, such as satisfaction with social support, are important. It is possible, however, that psychological distress may influence the perceived quality of social support and may reduce the quality of social interaction.

The above evidence describes how behavioural factors can influence our mood; the case example 'The relationship between mood and behaviour' puts this into context. Clearly, the relationship between behaviour and mood is complex; physiological, emotional and social influences have been proposed as **mediators** of the relationship. Whatever the cause and effect, the thoughts, feelings, behaviour and physiology cycle shown in Figure 2.1 is helpful in reminding us as clinicians that identifying and helping our clients to address unhelpful aspects of any of these elements is necessary to provide holistic and person-centred care.

Case Example: The relationship between mood and behaviour

Mark is 32 years old and has Down's Syndrome. He does not work and lives in a care home. Most evenings he visits the local pub. He is chatty, likes a good joke and is well known to the regulars who buy him drinks.

Mark enjoys drinking beer and the company of the other men in the pub, but the next day he often feels hungover and tired. He gets up late and often can't be bothered to do much, though most days one of his carers will persuade him to join them for a walk. Mark is quite overweight, and so is the carer, neither feel like walking far or fast.

Over time, Mark is becoming less and less fit so the walks, his only exercise, are becoming harder and less enjoyable for him. He is choosing to shorten his walks more each day.

At home he watches TV and snacks on unhealthy foods through boredom. Mark's weight is increasing and the only thing he looks forward to is going to the pub. However, lately he has sometimes felt too fed up to bother going out. When he has made it to the pub, he has been quieter than usual. The other regulars still buy him drinks, but spend less time in his company as he has become less fun to talk to. Visits to the pub have become less pleasurable for Mark so he is less and less motivated to make the effort to get there.

In Chapter 4 your will learn ways to help people like Mark make and sustain healthy choices which will also help to improve the person's mood.

DETECTING COMMON MENTAL DISORDERS

So far we have established that CMDs are common, that people with physical illness are at risk of developing them and that they are associated with worse outcome. CMDs are also strongly associated with suicide and are present in around 90 per cent of people who commit suicide: more than half of all suicides occur in people who meet the criteria for depression diagnosis (Hawton and van Heeringen, 2009). It is therefore important for us as nurses, midwives and health visitors to be able to recognise when patients are experiencing mood difficulties. This is especially so since patients may not ask directly for help due to embarrassment, stigma, lack of knowledge or worries about treatments. This may especially be the case in people with existing physical health problems, who may consider mood problems as 'to be expected' and may not understand that treatment is available. Older people or people of certain ethnicities may be particularly likely to feel that feelings of low or anxious mood are a sign of weakness and avoid seeking help. This attitude is known as 'self stigma' (Corrigan, 2004). The factors involved in assessing suicide risk are detailed in Box 2.3.

Box 2.3: Assessing risk of suicide and self-harm

Risk factors for suicide include: genetic loading, personality (impulsivity, aggression), restricted fetal growth and perinatal circumstances, early traumatic life events, neurobiological disturbances, psychiatric disorder, physical illness and disability, psychosocial crisis, availability of means and exposure to models (experience of other's suicide, directly or via the media). (From: Hawton and van Heeringen, 2009.) Drug and alcohol use and evidence or reports of self-harm may be important.

Assessment: Morriss et al. (2013) have produced an evidence-based guide for assessing risk of suicide and self-harm for non-mental health specialists. Essentially, the usual assessment process for CMD applies; in addition, risk factors should be considered and current thoughts (e.g. feelings of hopelessness, wishes to be dead), plans and intent should be explored, as these are associated with suicide attempts.

Management: If self-harm or suicidal intent is suspected, Morriss et al. (2013) recommend: drawing up a summary of risk to form a coherent narrative; discussing with colleagues or a mental health expert; making a plan based on the narrative summary (treatment decisions, referral, follow up, provide information on sources of help); end with engendering hope and summarising shared agreement for the plan.

A range of skills, resources and knowledge are needed to detect CMDs; these are outlined next.

Communication Skills

Excellent communication skills are needed to build sufficient trust for the patient to disclose difficult feelings. Displaying empathy and exploring the patient's expectations and preferences are essential to assessment and ongoing support (Maguire and Pitceathly, 2002). NICE guidance (NICE CG123, 2011b) is that 'all staff carrying out the assessment of common mental health disorders should be competent in relevant verbal and non-verbal communication skills, including the ability to elicit problems, the perception of the problem(s) and their impact, tailoring information, supporting participation in decision-making and discussing treatment options.'

Time

Pressures on our time are high, but time taken to identify factors important to ongoing management, such as past history of mental health problems, previous response to treatments, history of self-harm, and current suicidal ideas will save time in the long run by informing the most effective plan of care.

Awareness of Cultural and Social Factors

The presentation of CMDs may vary widely, and culture, age, social and educational factors can play an important part in patients' willingness to express problems and the types of complaints they share. For instance, people from non-Western cultures may be more likely to present with somatic (bodily) features of mental health problems (Bhugra and Mastrogianni, 2004). There are additional factors to consider when assessing mood in children and young people, women in the perinatal period and older adults; these are described in Box 2.4. Alcohol and drug use is associated with CMDs and patients should be asked about this.

Box 2.4: Detecting CMDs – special considerations

Children and young people

Risk factors include: long-term physical illness; a parent who has mental health problems, problems with alcohol or has been in trouble with the law; death of an important other; parental separation or divorce; being bullied or abused; living in poverty or being homeless; discrimination (due to race, sexuality or religion); having a carer or other adult responsibilities; long-standing educational difficulties (Mental Health Foundation, 2014). Assessment is complicated as children, and especially teenagers, may be uncommunicative and questionnaire measures may not be as reliable. Healthcare professionals should be alert to behavioural indicators of CMD such as impaired functioning at school or socially, bad behaviour, mood swings, self-harm or changes in eating patterns.

Women in the perinatal period

Risk factors for postnatal depression include: depressed mood and depression or anxiety during pregnancy; limited social support; recent adverse life events; past history of mental health problems. Healthcare professionals should assess pregnant women and new mothers for these risk factors. Generic measures of depression can be used; the Edinburgh Postnatal Depression Scale (Cox et al., 1987) is also available.

Older adults

Depression in the elderly may be perceived as due to ageing, but this is wrong (Burroughs et al., 2006); it is strongly associated with physical illness. When assessing for CMDs in the elderly, healthcare professionals should be aware that older depressed adults often present with somatic symptoms; they may be more likely than younger people to fear stigmatisation, believe that antidepressant medication is addictive, or to misattribute symptoms of major depression for 'old age', ill health or grief (Burroughs et al., 2006). Generic questionnaires may be used; the Geriatric Depression Scale (Koenig et al., 1988) has been validated for older adults in a range of settings. Depression in dementia is common and often missed (Kales et al., 2005). When assessing for CMDs in dementia, carers should be consulted.

Awareness of Clinical Features or Symptoms of CMD

Features of depression are listed in DSM-5. Nurses, midwives and health visitors should look out for these signs which include:

- low mood
- loss of interest and pleasure
- significant weight loss or gain
- physical agitation

- fatigue or loss of energy
- significant distress or impairment
- feelings of worthlessness or excessive guilt
- reduced concentration
- indecisiveness

According to DSM-5, excessive worry is the main symptom of anxiety disorders so we should assess further patients or relatives who appear to have a disproportionate or unusual number of concerns. Other cognitive or somatic symptoms of anxiety include:

- Cognitive:
  - angst
  - irritability
  - fear
  - difficulty concentrating
  - increased startle
  - hypervigilance
  - compulsions
  - obsessions

- Somatic:
  - restlessness
  - muscle tension
  - shortness of breath
  - sleep disturbance
  - easily fatigued
  - palpitations
  - choking

These symptoms are commonly experienced in normal daily life and do not necessarily indicate CMD. It is their intensity, duration and the extent to which they impair the person's ability to function that differentiates CMD from normal experience.

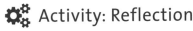 **Activity: Reflection**

Patients may tell you about these symptoms or you may infer some from their body language. Consider how you can detect signs of low mood or distress by observing them. List the signs you might see.

Screening Instruments – Depression

Several self-report instruments exist. Two items derived from the core features of depression (DSM-5) are a simple assessment tool. Named the 'Whooley questions' after the researcher who initially tested the effect of these (Whooley et al., 1997), these two simple items provide correct identification in 95 per cent of people who have depression (high *sensitivity*). Patients are asked to respond Yes or No to:

1. During the past month, have you often been bothered by feeling down, depressed, or hopeless?
2. During the past month, have you often been bothered by little interest or pleasure in doing things?

A positive response to either or both identifies a person as having possible depression.

However, only 66 per cent of people (low *specificity*) who do *not* have depression will be correctly recognised as non-cases by these two questions (NICE, 2009a); that is, a significant number of people will be falsely identified as depressed. Following a positive response, further assessment is therefore necessary to determine whether or not the person is depressed.

Hence, the questions are often presented as part of a longer instrument – the PHQ-9 (Kroenke et al., 2001). Seven subsequent questions assess the type and number of symptoms that the person is experiencing, their severity and duration and their effects on daily life, and is based upon the DSM-5 diagnostic criteria. It is widely used in the UK in clinical practice and in research, is brief and simple to complete, and has good sensitivity and specificity for depression alone and co-morbid with medical problems (NICE, 2009a, 2009b). A score of 10 or above will correctly identify 82 per cent of depressed patients in healthcare settings, while 83 per cent of people of non-cases will score below 10 (NICE, 2009a).

Similarly valid (NICE, 2009a) alternative instruments are available including: the Beck Depression Inventory (BDI) (Beck et al., 1961); the Hospital Anxiety and Depression Scale (HADS) (Zigmond and Snaith, 1983); the Center for Epidemiological Studies Depression Scale (CES-D) (Radloff, 1977); and the Geriatric Depression Scale (GDS-15) (Yesavage et al., 1982). However, these other instruments are longer and some (the BDI and HADS) are subject to copyright restrictions, which means they are not free to use.

Screening Instruments – Anxiety

Similar to the PHQ-2 for depression, the Generalised Anxiety Disorder Assessment 2 (GAD-2) consists of two items, which are taken from a longer seven-item questionnaire – the GAD-7 – which was devised in 2006 by Spitzer and colleagues (2006) to detect generalised anxiety disorder.

Patients are asked: Over the past two weeks, how often have you been bothered by:

1. Feeling nervous, anxious or on edge?
2. Not being able to stop or control worrying?

There is a choice of four response options: Not at all, several days, more than half the days, or nearly every day. People scoring a combined score of 3 or more are considered potentially to be suffering from an anxiety disorder.

These questions may not detect anxiety associated with phobia; therefore, if you suspect an anxiety problem but the individual scores less than 3, a further question:

'Do you find yourself avoiding places/activities and does this cause you problems?', should also be asked.

The GAD-2 has been found to work almost as well in detecting anxiety disorders as the longer GAD-7; sensitivity is particularly good for generalised anxiety disorder, which is unsurprising, but it is also good for panic disorder and social anxiety disorder and to a slightly lesser extent PTSD (Kroenke et al., 2007). The additional five questions of the GAD-7 may be useful in clinical practice when we want to grade severity or monitor change over time as they provide a wider scoring range.

Detecting CMDs in People with Low Literacy Levels

Items from short questionnaires like the PHQ-9 or GAD-7 can be read aloud to patients, though this may inhibit some people responding. A pictorial 'distress thermometer', where the person is asked to mark a line labelled from no distress to extreme distress, or a selection of pictures of faces showing a range of emotions may be more appropriate for some. Alternatively, carer or relatives may provide information about the individual's mental state.

DETECTING CMDs – SUMMARY

Simply administering an instrument and checking symptoms is insufficient for assessing a mental health problem. Healthcare professionals need to use their communication skills, including their knowledge of non-verbal communication, to determine the severity and impact of troublesome emotion. Past history of mental health problems and treatments should be reviewed and current stressors and sources of support considered. Risk factors for specific populations should be considered and risk of self-harm or suicide assessed.

MANAGING TROUBLESOME EMOTION

Effective Communication

Effective communication is essential for all aspects of care assessment, planning, implementation and evaluation. Communication can be hindered in the presence of troublesome emotion in a number of ways. For instance, we have discussed above how troublesome emotion may be associated with thinking errors: patients who are feeling hopeless may lack **motivation** to follow treatment regimens; stressed or anxious patients may be overly concerned about the side effects of medications; angry people may have unreasonable expectations of care. Troublesome emotion can be so consuming that highly stressed, angry or grieving people may be unable to understand and process new information. Written, evidence-based information tailored to the patient's needs and which is culturally appropriate and accessible is useful for patients to take away so that they can refer to it in their own time and at their own pace.

Effective Communication Behaviours

Clinician behaviours are important for effective communication. Making these explicit will help alert you to your own helpful and unhelpful habits.

 Activity: Reflection

Make a list of behaviours that you know help or hinder communication with patients (and/or colleagues!). Some examples are provided at the end of the chapter.

Essentially, unhelpful behaviours undermine patients and prevent effective **shared decision-making**. Helpful behaviours help patients to process and understand information and make them feel valued and empowered. This increases self-efficacy and motivation and hence the likelihood of advice or treatment regimens being carried out.

Helpful behaviours also contribute to the development of a good therapeutic relationship, which contributes to patient engagement with services; this may be particularly the case for people living with severe mental illness (Priebe et al., 2005; Kirsch and Tate, 2006). In the delivery of psychological therapy, a meta-analysis of 79 studies indicated that a good therapeutic relationship (also known as a helping/ working or therapeutic alliance) is an essential factor in the efficacy of treatment (Martin et al., 2000a). We will consider the application of helpful communication behaviours to specific clinical situations in Chapters 5 and 6.

MANAGING HEIGHTENED EMOTION

Effective communication skills are nowhere more important than in situations where emotions are running high, for instance, when patients, or their relatives, are angry or agitated. Verbal 'de-escalation techniques' have been developed to help manage agitated patients in mental health settings to avoid the use of restraint and involuntary medication (Richmond et al., 2012). In such situations, agitation is an acute behavioural emergency and an adequate number of appropriately trained staff is needed for safe use of the techniques. However, the general principles can be applied in other settings where emotions may be getting out of hand but are less immediately 'explosive'.

The aim of de-escalation is to help the person to calm themselves (as opposed to 'calming the patient down' which has a dominant-submissive connotation), in order that they can re-establish their own internal locus of control (Richmond et al., 2012). Fishkind (2002) has suggested ten 'domains of de-escalation'; these are shown in Table 2.1. Richmond et al. (2012) build on these and propose a 3-stage approach where 1) the patient is verbally engaged; 2) a collaborative relationship is established; 3) the patient is verbally de-escalated out of the agitated state.

Table 2.1 Ten domains of de-escalation

Respect personal space

Do not be provocative

Establish verbal contact

Be concise

Identify wants and feelings

Listen closely to what the patient is saying

Agree or agree to disagree

Lay down the law and set clear limits

Offer choices and optimism

Debrief the patient and staff

From: Fishkind (2002) and Richmond et al. (2012) by permission of the Publisher

TREATMENT OF CMDs

When working with people who have a CMD, NICE stresses the importance of person-centred care, which takes into account patients' needs and preferences. Treatment for CMD follows a stepped care approach where the least intrusive, most effective intervention is provided first; if a person does not benefit from the first treatment or declines it, they are offered an intervention from the next step. Which interventions are available will vary by area and local policies may differ. It is important to familiarise yourself with the options available to your patients; examples are provided in Table 2.2.

Table 2.2 Example stepped care interventions for CMDs

Step	Example intervention
Step 1: Possible CMD	Identification and assessment, psycho-education, active monitoring, if you do not feel competent to perform a mental health assessment, refer the person to an appropriate professional
Step 2: Persistent subthreshold depressive symptoms; mild to moderate depression; diagnosed GAD that has not improved after education and active monitoring in primary care	Low intensity intervention, e.g. guided self-help, computerised CBT, structured exercise programme, peer support group, non-directive counselling, psychosocial intervention, group psychoeducation

(Continued)

Table 2.2 (Continued)

Step	Example intervention
Step 3: Persistent subthreshold depressive symptoms; mild to moderate CMDs or GAD with inadequate response to initial interventions; moderate to severe CMDs; marked functional impairment	Medication (e.g. antidepressant, anxiolytic) and/or evidence-based high intensity psychological therapy, e.g. CBT, interpersonal therapy, behavioural activation or behavioural couples therapy, or, for people who refused these, counselling or short-term psychodynamic psychotherapy, though discussion around lack of evidence for the effectiveness of these therapies in depression should be undertaken, applied relaxation
Step 4: Severe and complex depression; risk to life; complex treatment-refractory GAD; very marked functional impairment, such as self-neglect or a high risk of self-harm	Medication, high-intensity psychological interventions, electroconvulsive therapy, crisis service, combined treatments, multiprofessional and inpatient care

Adapted with permission from NICE (2011b) and available from www.nice.org.uk/CG123

CHAPTER SUMMARY

Common mental disorders (CMDs) have been described and their detection and management explored. Evidence for predictors, such as gender, ethnicity, medical history, child birth and alcohol misuse, was presented.

How the concepts of stress, anger and grief are understood by health psychologists was explored. A distinction was made between normal and troublesome emotion.

CMDs and stress, anger and grief can have a negative impact on physical and mental health. The pathways for this are unclear, but may be physiological, behavioural or cognitive.

How thoughts, feelings, physiology and behaviour interact was explored. Unhelpful beliefs or thinking errors can lead to distress. If identified by healthcare professionals they can be modified or replaced by more helpful cognitions.

Healthcare professionals need a range of resources and skills, including communication skills, awareness of cultural and social factors and knowledge of symptoms and screening instruments, to be able to detect troublesome emotion and help patients to manage its impact on health.

CONSOLIDATE YOUR LEARNING

 Activity: Quiz

(Answers can be found at the end of this book.)

1. How long should symptoms have been present before a diagnosis of depression can be made?
2. List some known predictors of common mental disorders.

3. Does physical illness cause CMDs or do CMDs lead to physical illness?
4. According to cognitive theories, what four interacting factors should we consider when assessing or managing patients?

⚙ Activity: Reflection

Using health psychology to help patients manage troublesome emotion

- Consider one of your patients. How do their emotions impact on their condition?
- Are they experiencing a normal or a troublesome level of emotion?
- What tools could you use to find out?
- Have you noticed the kind of thoughts they are experiencing about their condition?
- Could they be making any 'thinking errors' and, if so, could you suggest more helpful ways of thinking?

FURTHER READING

Stress: Hill Rice, V. (2012) *Handbook of Stress, Coping, and Health Implications for Nursing Research, Theory, and Practice* (Second edition). London: Sage.
Depression: Haddad, M. and Gunn, J. (2011). *Fast Facts: Depression* (Third revised edition). Abingdon: Health Press Limited.

USEFUL WEBSITES

Grief: The National Cancer Institute in the USA has produced a comprehensive review of grief research – www.cancer.gov/cancertopics/pdq/supportivecare/bereavement/HealthProfessional/page3
Cognitive Behavioural Therapy: Beck Institute Blog – www.beckinstitute.org/

Relevant NICE guidance:

NICE CG16 (2004) Self-harm in over 8s: longer-term management. www.nice.org.uk/guidance/cg16
NICE CG90 (2009) Depression in adults: recognition and management. www.nice.org.uk/guidance/cg90
NICE CG28 (2005) Depression in children and young people: identification and management. www.nice.org.uk/guidance/cg28
NICE CG113 (2011) Generalised anxiety disorder and panic disorder in adults. www.nice.org.uk/guidance/cg113
NICE CG123 (2011) Common mental health disorders: identification and pathways to care. www.nice.org.uk/guidance/cg123
NICE CG91 (2009) Depression in adults with a chronic physical health problem: recognition and management. www.nice.org.uk/guidance/cg91

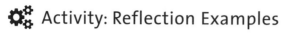

Activity: Reflection Examples

p. 22 Examples of factors which may influence perceptions of threat and ability to cope: previous experience, perceived resources, habits, feelings of self-efficacy, locus of control, illness beliefs, availability of information, controllability of the situation, finances and availability of social support, etc.

p. 38 Examples of behaviours that help or hinder communication:

Helpful	Unhelpful
Active listening	Use of jargon
Appropriate use of open and closed questions	Being judgemental
Providing verbal information summaries – clarifying points, reflecting statements and feelings, ascertaining understanding	Being patronising
Demonstrating empathy	Being distracted – e.g. answering the telephone or focusing on typing on a computer during a consultation
Body language – relaxed, open posture, eye contact	Body language – tense, rushed, avoiding eye contact
Providing affirmations/encouragement	Interrupting

3 IMPROVING SELF-MANAGEMENT

Key Learning Objectives

At the end of this chapter you will be able to explain:

- What a long-term condition is
- Management and self-management of long-term conditions
- Factors which support self-management, including **self-efficacy** and **social support**
- Illness perceptions and their impact on self-management
- Treatment adherence, including unintentional and intentional contributing factors

INTRODUCTION

This chapter will address how healthcare professionals can best support their patients to self-manage their conditions. Tools useful for nurses, midwives and health visitors to support self-management will be described and the evidence for their use discussed. The focus in this chapter will be on the management of long-term conditions, in particular on helping people to follow treatment regimens. How **health psychology** helps us to help people to make healthy choices in general and to cope with common symptoms, which are also important aspects of self-management, will be discussed in later chapters, though much of what is discussed here will be relevant to these situations.

LONG-TERM CONDITIONS

Most research around self-management has focused on long-term conditions (LTCs). These are conditions which cannot be cured, but which can be managed with medication and/or other treatments including lifestyle changes; the need for self-management is therefore ongoing. Non-communicable LTCs include asthma, chronic obstructive pulmonary disease (COPD), coronary heart disease (CHD), diabetes, hypertension, arthritis, chronic kidney disease, epilepsy and many more.

Increasingly, due to improved survival rates, cancer is managed as a LTC. Infectious diseases such as HIV and tuberculosis also require long-term self-management, as do some mental health conditions such as psychotic disorders and depression in its **chronic**, remitting and relapsing and treatment resistant forms. Many **medically unexplained syndromes**, such as irritable bowel syndrome, **chronic fatigue syndrome, fibromyalgia** and chronic low back pain, are also enduring.

In England, about 30 per cent of the population have one or more LTCs and they account for about 70 per cent of total spending on health and care (DH, 2012). Many people have more than one LTC and rates of this '**multimorbidity**' are increasing with an expected rise to 2.9 million in 2018 from 1.9 million in 2008 (DH, 2012). LTCs are associated with inequality as there are higher rates of many LTCs in those from lower socio-economic groups, and the onset of multimorbidity has been found to occur 10–15 years earlier among those living in deprived areas (Coulter et al., 2013). LTCs have considerable impact on an individual's ability to work and to lead a full life. Impact on quality of life may result from a combination of symptoms, loss of function and independence and strain on personal relationships. As discussed in Chapter 2, LTCs are also associated with increased prevalence of psychological distress (Moussavi et al., 2007).

⚙ Activity Answers: Reflection

As you read through the following sections, consider the implications of 'multimorbidity' for your patients, their dependents or their carers and for healthcare delivery. How many of your patients have more than one LTC? Which conditions often co-occur and why?

In what way is multimorbidity more than just the sum of the single conditions? Consider interactions between symptoms and treatments, implications for screening, diagnosis and management in the context of care pathways designed for single conditions.

MANAGEMENT OF LTCs

For many LTCs, lifestyle and ageing are important for both their development and impact. Management goals are around prevention, delaying onset, reducing exacerbations and slowing progression. The aim is to improve quality of life for the patient. Achieving value for money in care is also important, effective self-management may also reduce unscheduled hospital admissions which are costly, but also distressing and disrupting for patients and their families (70 per cent of inpatient bed days in England are due to LTCs; DH, 2012). Unnecessary GP attendances may also be avoided; for instance, for symptoms such as chest pain, palpitations, breathlessness and fatigue, which are commonly chronic and for which further physical treatment is often unavailable (see Chapter 5 for health psychology interventions for managing these symptoms).

The burden of managing LTCs on health services is great; there is also huge burden on patients and their carers who have to manage treatment regimens, including medications and self-monitoring (for instance, blood glucose testing in people with diabetes) and organise and co-ordinate healthcare appointments, including visits to GPs, practice nurses, hospital clinics and for tests (such as blood tests); those who need social care will also have to negotiate welfare agencies and, in countries without a National Health Service, patients will need to contend with the demands of insurance agencies (May et al., 2009). From review evidence, it appears that both patients and informal carers may spend two hours a day or more on health-related activities associated with LTCs (Jowsey et al., 2012). Patients and their carers therefore need a range of skills and resources to manage their LTC(s).

Self-management

Self-management has been defined as 'the individual's ability to manage the symptoms, treatment, physical and psychosocial consequences and lifestyle changes inherent in living with a chronic condition' (Barlow et al., 2002). This definition emphasises that skills (for instance, being able to read a prescription) and resources (for example, access to a means of travel to healthcare appointments) are necessary for self-management. Another definition that self-management is 'about people taking responsibility for their own health and **wellbeing**. It includes staying fit and healthy, taking action to prevent illness and accidents, using medicines effectively, treating minor ailments appropriately, and seeking professional help when necessary' (DH, 2009: 4) emphasises the personal responsibility of the patient for taking care of themselves. In the case of parents or carers, responsibility may be for a child or other dependent person (DH, 2005). Both definitions highlight the complexity of living with and coping with a LTC and it is well recognised that people need support to self-manage.

Self-management support is 'about supporting people in the decisions they make to manage their LTC. It is also about offering individuals the right information and support at the right time, and empowering them to take a more active role in their health and wellbeing in order to improve their quality of life' (DH, 2009: 4). Self-management support is most effective when there is **shared decision-making** – that is when a patient and their healthcare professional make choices around healthcare together, taking into account what is important to each person. An example of this is shown in the case example 'Shared decision-making in diabetes'. Knowledge of health psychology can help nurses, midwives and health visitors to discover what is important to patients, identify and overcome barriers to self-management, identify and utilise facilitators to self-management, present information about self-management in a way that patients can understand and help boost people's confidence and understanding of their responsibility to manage their own health.

Self-management support increases patient activation; patients who are more 'activated' tend to have better outcomes (Hibbard and Greene, 2013). For instance, a cross-sectional study conducted in the USA (Greene and Hibbard, 2012) of 25,047 adults found that more activated patients had better clinical indicators (HbA1c, HDL, triglycerides), were more likely to have received preventive care (breast cancer screen), and were less likely to smoke, to have a high BMI, to have been hospitalised or to have visited an emergency department. There is a growing body of research which shows that patient levels of activation can be modified and increased over time and effective interventions for building activation have been developed (Hibbard and Greene, 2013).

Case Example: Shared decision-making in diabetes

Noreen is a 62-year-old woman with a **body mass index** of 26.4, which means she is overweight. She has just been diagnosed with type 2 diabetes; her GP has prescribed Metformin. Noreen also has long-standing asthma, which is well controlled using a Pulmicort (budesonide) turbohaler twice daily and ventolin very occasionally.

At her annual asthma check a week later, Noreen confides to her practice nurse that she has not been using the Metformin. The nurse takes time to understand Noreen's reasons for not taking the medication. These seem to revolve around a fear that long-term medications are 'bad for you' (see '**illness perceptions**' on p. 50). The nurse is able to provide health education about the safety and efficacy of Metformin. She also highlights how Noreen's long-term medication for her asthma has helped her.

She then discusses treatment options (do nothing; make lifestyle changes; take medication) and explores the pros and cons of each with Noreen. The nurse checks that Noreen understands all this information. Noreen agrees a course of action with the nurse. She decides that she will take the Metformin as prescribed as she knows from past experience that it will be too difficult to make the necessary lifestyle changes quickly enough.

The nurse schedules another appointment to see how Noreen is getting on with the tablets and to discuss making lifestyle changes in the longer term.

Promoting Effective Self-management

Decision Aids

Decision aids are information resources (pamphlet, video, web-based tool) that help people to work with their healthcare professional to make healthcare choices. They are designed to help people to weigh up the pros and cons of different choices and to help them to understand what is important to them. They therefore support shared decision-making. In the above case example, the practice nurse could have used a decision aid to structure her consultation with Noreen. Decision aids have been developed for a range of conditions (see Useful Websites below) and healthcare situations. A Cochrane review of decision aids for people facing health treatment or screening decisions (Stacey et al., 2014) identified 115 RCTs (total N=34,444) comparing decision aids with usual care or an alternative. The review found high-quality evidence that decision aids improve people's knowledge of options and reduce their decisional conflict. It also found moderate-quality evidence that decision aids help people to be more active in their decision-making and that, when probabilities are included in decision aids, they improve the accuracy of risk perceptions. Low-quality evidence was found that decision aids improve the match between the option chosen and the patient's **values**. Recent evidence identified by the reviews found that decision aids were associated with more informed, values-based choices and improved patient-practitioner communication, though the effect on length of consultation varied. Consistent with findings from the previous review, decision aids have a variable effect on choices. More research is needed to determine the best form of decision aid and differential effects on different populations.

Self-management Education

Self-management education programmes are 'distinct from simple patient education or skills training, in that they are designed to allow people with chronic conditions to take an active part in the management of their own condition' (Foster et al., 2007). Systematic reviews of self-management education programmes have tended to find small to moderate effects (Warsi et al., 2004). Such programmes may be led by healthcare professionals or by lay people (known as expert patients). A Cochrane review of 17 studies (total N=7442) of lay-led self-management education in people with arthritis, diabetes, hypertension and chronic pain (Foster et al., 2007) found evidence for small, short-term improvements in participants' self-efficacy, self-rated health, cognitive symptom management, and frequency of aerobic exercise. Similarly, an evaluation of the UK Government's expert patient programme, which included an RCT (n=629 patients with a range of LTCs) comparing a six-week programme with a waiting list condition, found improvements in self-efficacy and energy levels, and evidence of cost effectiveness.

A difficulty in reviewing the evidence for self-management education programmes is that across studies the programmes may contain different elements and may therefore not be comparable; some elements may be more effective than others. Programmes may to a greater or lesser extent include passive information provision and teaching of 'technical skills' (e.g. blood glucose testing) or elements that more actively promote behaviour change (e.g. psychological interventions) (de Silva, 2011).

The Role of Self-efficacy in Self-management

A comprehensive systematic review conducted by the Health Foundation (de Silva, 2011) of over 550 high-quality studies of a range of interventions to support self-management indicates that building **self-efficacy** is key and that interventions which do so have a positive effect on clinical symptoms and outcomes, **attitudes** and behaviours, quality of life, and use of healthcare resources. Unfortunately, the authors conclude that the best strategies for increasing self-efficacy are unknown. Self-efficacy theory (Bandura, 1977) predicts that an individual's self-efficacy arises from four main sources: performance accomplishments, vicarious experience, social persuasion and physiological and emotional responses. The most important source is likely to vary by population and situation, but interventions which influence these sources would be predicted to increase self-efficacy.

Sources of Self-efficacy

Performance accomplishments – also known as '**mastery experiences**' are personal experiences of achievement or success in a particular task or situation, and may be the strongest predictor of self-efficacy. Repeated success will increase 'mastery expectation', i.e. the individual's belief that they will be successful in future similar situations. Healthcare professionals can help increase their patients' mastery expectations by helping patients faced with difficult challenges to recall past successes in similar situations. For instance, if a patient is struggling to cope with pain, reminding them of, or asking them to remember, past occasions when they have coped and, in particular, which coping strategies they used that were successful, can be very powerful in helping them to cope in the current situation.

Vicarious experience – also referred to as 'social modelling', involves observing others successfully performing a task. This builds self-efficacy by generating expectations in the individual observing the successful performance that they too can succeed by applying what they have learnt from their observations. Opportunities to observe others coping with similar difficulties to their own can be provided by 'expert patients' or 'peer supporters' (see below).

Social persuasion – this refers to helping an individual believe they can succeed with a particular task. This may be achieved through the provision of encouragement by family, significant others or healthcare professionals or by more formal evaluative feedback, where specific positive aspects of an individual's performance are highlighted. Such techniques are used in health coaching which can also be used a means of social persuasion to promote self-efficacy (Box 3.1).

Physiological and emotional responses – an individual's mental or bodily response to a situation or task will influence their belief in their ability to manage the situation or achieve the task. For instance, anxiety around attending for hospital tests make may the patients less likely to attend. It can be helpful for healthcare professionals to talk through specific anxieties with patients; reassurance may be provided or strategies for overcoming barriers derived. For instance, explaining to a patient how their pain will be managed during a procedure may reassure them that they will be able to endure it.

Box 3.1: Health coaching

Definition: health coaching is a formal, structured conversation with a client which involves 'applying skills of listening, questioning and reflecting to support persons with a chronic illness to manage the physical, psychological and social influences of the disease' (Howard and Ceci, 2013: 225).

Coaching differs from traditional education provision as, rather than giving advice and direction, a coach's role is to ask powerful questions designed to help the individual to find their own answers.

Coaching emphasises that sustained efforts and commitment are required for a successful outcome (Neenan and Dryden, 2002).

Self-efficacy may be enhanced by using coaching skills to promote a patient's belief that they can succeed at a task or cope in a difficult situation (social persuasion) and by encouraging recall of past success (mastery experiences).

Evidence – A review of 15 RCTs of health coaching interventions found significant improvements in one or more of healthy eating, physical activity, weight management and medication adherence in six of the studies. The quality of the included studies varied, as did the content of the interventions; common features of those that were effective were goal setting (see Chapter 4), motivational interviewing (see Chapter 4), and collaboration with healthcare providers.

The Role of Social Support in Self-management

Social support – help available from others – is an important resource for promoting self-management. It is essential for the wellbeing of patients and their carers; for instance, in families experiencing stressful circumstances social support has been found to protect against harmful effects of stress, but also to have beneficial effects on wellbeing whether or not the person is currently under stress (Armstrong et al., 2005). As well as helping with the stress of illness, social support facilitates self-management through providing motivation and encouragement and help with problem solving. A review (Gallant, 2003) of 29 studies (mostly of diabetes, but also asthma, heart disease and epilepsy) found evidence for a modest positive relationship between social support and LTC self-management. However, the process by which social support influences self-management and whether the relationship varies by illness, type of support and behaviour could not be determined. A later study of 2,572 patients with type 2 diabetes (Schiøtz et al., 2012) found that seeing friends and family more frequently, having a well-functioning **social network** and a sense of good social support from the social network were associated with better outcomes and improved self-management. A poor functional social network, measured as perceived lack of help in the event of severe illness, was associated with worse outcomes. This study highlights the importance of the quality (actual and perceived) of social support, as opposed to simply its availability. It can be useful to ask patients to identify individuals who can help them (Michie et al., 2008) and in what ways; this gives the patient a sense of control and a specific resource on which to draw in particular circumstances.

In the context of social cognition theory, social networks (interpersonal relationships) are also likely to influence self-management through **social norms** and values; for instance, around expectations of the extent of individual responsibility for one's own health. Relatively recently researchers have argued that current interventions to improve self-management are too focused on individual behaviour and that the role of social networks and **social capital** (the total amount of social resources available to an individual) should be emphasised (Vassilev et al., 2011). Different social support may be relevant for helping with different aspects of LTC management. Vassilev et al. (2013) separate the work of LTC management into: 'illness work', e.g. taking medications, recording vital signs, making appointments; 'everyday work', e.g. housekeeping, childcare, shopping; and 'emotional work', e.g. providing comfort when depressed or anxious. Healthcare professionals could ask patients to identify individuals who can help with each of these aspects.

A special example of a social support intervention is '**peer support**' where support is provided to patients or carers by people with a similar condition to the patient or with experience of caring for someone with a similar condition. Usually a peer supporter has had some kind of training or is more experienced in managing the condition than the person they are supporting (Burnell et al., 2012). Benefits are thought to be that support is perceived as grounded in experiential knowledge and is specific to a particular condition, circumstance or cultural setting (Doull et al., 2005); this specialist knowledge provides the 'expert' with credibility. Peer support interventions have been tested in a range of long-term physical and mental conditions, in adults and children, though evidence for their effectiveness is inconsistent and a full systematic review is needed (Doull et al., 2005). A meta-synthesis of 25 qualitative studies of people's experience of peer support interventions for a range of LTCs (Embuldeniya et al., 2013) identified both positive and negative effects; for instance, sharing of experience facilitated communication and rapport, but it could also foster a competitive culture of 'whose condition was worse'.

The Role of Illness Perceptions in Self-management

In Chapter 1, evidence was presented showing how health beliefs, as specified by health psychology **models** such as the Health Belief Model (Rosenstock, 1966; Becker, 1974) and the Theory of Reasoned Action (Fishbein and Ajzen, 1975) may predict health behaviour. In Chapter 2, we considered how thoughts, feelings and behaviours are linked according to cognitive models (Beck, 1967). Here we consider how specific beliefs about illness, or 'illness perceptions', may impact on self-management.

The Common-Sense Model of Self-Regulation of Health and Illness (Leventhal et al., 1980, 2003) was proposed to explain this. The model proposes five dimensions of illness perceptions: cause, identity (the symptoms or impacts that the patient sees as related to their illness), perceived control (treatment-related and personal), severity of illness consequences and timeline (see Box 3.2 for examples of illness perceptions related to these dimensions). Subsequent health psychology research has added further dimensions of 'illness coherence', a belief that the illness 'makes sense' to the patient, 'emotional representations', how the illness makes the person feel, and 'cyclical timeline' which is useful in conditions where effects come and go (Moss-Morris et al., 2002).

Illness perceptions guide coping actions and influence emotional outcomes such as illness-related distress (Hagger and Orbell, 2003). They have also been found to be implicated in self-management behaviour; for instance, in a study of 93 people invited to attend cardiac rehabilitation (Whitmarsh et al., 2003), attenders compared with poor/non-attenders perceived that they had a greater number of symptoms and consequences of their illness and had less strong beliefs that their illness had been caused by a germ or virus, they were also more distressed and used problem-focused and emotion-focused coping more frequently. The best predictors of poor/non-attendance were lower perceived symptoms and controllability/curability of illness, as well as less frequent use of problem-focused and more frequent use of maladaptive coping strategies.

> # Box 3.2: Illness perceptions and potential impacts, categorised using the dimensions proposed by the Common-sense Model of Self-regulation of Health and Illness (Leventhal et al., 1980, 2003; Moss-Morris, 2002).
>
> Causal – 'My COPD is caused by God's will.' Potential impact: the patient feels like a victim and lacks motivation to engage in treatment.
>
> Identity – 'My angina prevents me from doing anything.' Potential impact: the patient limits their activity more than they need.
>
> Perceived control (treatment-related) – 'My medication doesn't help.' Potential impact: the patient stops taking their prescribed medication.
>
> Perceived control (personal) – 'Nothing I do will make my diabetes better.' Potential impact: the patient loses motivation to eat healthily.
>
> Severity of illness consequences – 'I have to give up work because of my heart disease, I won't be able to pay my mortgage and I will lose my house.' Potential impact: the patient's anxiety is hugely increased.
>
> Timeline – (**acute**/chronic) 'This pain will never go away.' Potential impact: the patient loses hope, becomes distressed.
>
> Timeline – (cyclical) 'I don't understand why I feel well some days and really bad on other days.' Potential impact: unable to predict 'well days' the patient finds it hard to plan activities and limits what they do.
>
> Emotional representations – 'I am so angry that I have cancer.' Potential impact: increased emotional distress.
>
> It should be noted that the same illness perception may have different effects in different individuals and may be held by an individual more or less strongly over time.

Much research focuses on unhelpful or negative illness perceptions, but illness perceptions can also be positive (e.g. reports of improved lifestyle, personal relationships and stress-reduction following diagnosis). Such perceptions, which are not associated with illness severity, have been found in patients following **myocardial infarction** or breast cancer diagnosis (Petrie et al., 1999) and in primary care patients living with a diagnosis of CHD (Smith et al., 2014). There is some evidence that positive illness perceptions or '**benefit finding**' may be beneficial to health. A systematic review of 77 studies in a range of conditions found benefit finding to be associated with less depression and better wellbeing, although it was also associated with more intrusive and avoidant thoughts about the stressor (Helgeson et al., 2006). Further research is needed to develop and test interventions which utilise positive illness perceptions to improve self-management, but nurses, midwives and health visitors may wish to help patients to identify any perceived positive effects of their condition or situation as a means of encouraging adaptation and emotional adjustment (Smith et al., 2014).

The Role of Telehealth in Self-management

The application of technology in healthcare is variously referred to as telehealth, telecare, telemedicine or ehealth. Telehealth interventions include electronic patient records, use of the internet or telephone lines for delivering interventions, remote monitoring and information sharing. Telehealth supports self-management by facilitating people to maintain independence and avoid unnecessary hospitalisation; for instance, remote monitoring of intrathoracic impedance, measured from an implanted device, can alert nurses to increases in pulmonary fluid retention in patients with heart failure and ensure timely intervention. Online interventions have been designed to support self-management in a variety of conditions by facilitating self-monitoring and providing psychoeducation or therapy (e.g. diabetes – Pal et al., 2013; asthma – Marcano Belisario et al., 2013; CVD – Barley et al., 2014; depression – Proudfoot et al., 2003). Such interventions are potentially easy to access, non-stigmatising (people can access them privately) and cost effective. Systematic reviews have found evidence of effectiveness, but online interventions tend to be multi-model and difficult to compare due to differences in content and purpose; the extent of the theoretical underpinning of different interventions also varies and this may impact on effectiveness (Marcano Belisario et al., 2013).

TREATMENT ADHERENCE

The extent to which patients follow treatment regimens agreed on with their healthcare providers (i.e. 'adherence' see Box 3.3) is highly predictive of outcome in LTCs, so understanding how to promote treatment adherence is important for all healthcare professionals. Effective medications exist for most LTCs, but many patients either stop taking them altogether or do not take them as prescribed. Medication adherence across LTCs is considered to average at around 50 per cent, with no significant change in the past half century (Nieuwlaat et al., 2014). In a review of 569 studies (DiMatteo, 2004) considering adherence to a range of physician recommendations (e.g. medications and behavioural changes) average non-adherence was found to be 25 per cent.

Box 3.3: Treatment adherence definitions

The following is adapted from Horne et al., 2006:

Compliance – 'The extent to which the patient's behaviour matches the prescriber's recommendations.' This definition implies lack of patient involvement and hence its use is declining.

Adherence – 'The extent to which the patient's behaviour matches agreed recommendations from the prescriber.' This term is used increasingly as it develops the definition of compliance by emphasising the need for agreement between patient and healthcare provider. It emphasises that the patient is free to decide whether to adhere to the doctor's recommendations and that failure to do so should not be a reason to blame the patient.

Another term, 'concordance', has been used relatively recently. This initially 'focused on the consultation process, in which doctor and patient agree therapeutic decisions that incorporate their respective views' and later has been used to refer to 'a wider concept which stretches from prescribing communication to patient support in medicine taking'.

Poor adherence has been shown in numerous studies (e.g. Ho et al., 2008; Sokol et al., 2005; Rasmussen et al., 2007; Dragomir et al., 2010) to be associated with adverse effects for patients including increased mortality, more hospitalisation, and the need for more expensive intervention and extended hospitalisation due to deterioration of conditions. Wasted resources and increased use of services place a cost burden on society.

UNDERSTANDING NON-ADHERENCE

Early research focused on identifying characteristics of conditions or individuals, which may predict non-compliance. Findings from this work made it clear that there is no such thing as a typical non-adherent patient (Horne, 2006); for instance, adherence is not related to disease type or severity, age, gender or socioeconomic status (DiMatteo, 2004; Horne, 2006), although there is some evidence that when the patient is paying for the medication, income is correlated (Piette et al., 2004).

More recently, understanding has increased that adherence represents a complex set of behaviours which may vary within the individual according to circumstance: people may adhere to all, some or no aspects of any treatment regimen at any given time. This, of course, makes an individual's behaviour hard to predict. The 'perceptions and practicalities model' (Horne, 2006) deconstructs the concept of adherence in an attempt to identify specific factors which may be addressed to prompt adherence. The model suggests that non-adherence can be considered as 'unintentional' or 'intentional'.

Unintentional non-adherence: with this type of non-adherence, the patient may be willing to take the prescribed medicines, or to make recommended behaviour changes, but they are prevented by either external or internal factors over which they may have little control. External factors include inadequate finance or lack of access to pharmacy. Internal factors include memory problems, chaotic or unmanageable lifestyle, inadequate comprehension of instructions, poor **health literacy** (Box 3.4) or physical inability to manage medications (e.g. poor inhaler technique (Horne, 2006)).

Box 3.4: Health literacy

Definition: More than a measure of achievement in reading and writing skills, health literacy has been defined as representing 'the cognitive and social skills which determine the motivation and ability of individuals to gain access to, understand and use information in ways which promote and maintain good health.' (Nutbeam, 1998: 357).

The WHO states that health literacy means more than being able to read pamphlets and successfully make appointments. By improving people's access to health information and their capacity to use it effectively, health literacy is critical to empowerment (WHO, 2015).

The evidence: 61 per cent of England's working-age population have low health literacy and those with the lowest levels of health literacy have the least access to health information – the 'inverse information law' (Rowlands and Nutbeam, 2013). A systematic review (n=111 studies) found that low health literacy was associated with more hospitalisations, greater use of emergency care, lower receipt of mammography screening and influenza vaccine, poorer ability to demonstrate taking medications appropriately, poorer ability to interpret labels and health messages, and, among elderly persons, poorer overall health status and higher mortality rates; poor health literacy also partially explained racial disparities in some outcomes (Berkman et al., 2011).

Health literacy is also important for child health. A systematic review (n=14 studies) found that children with low health literacy had worse health behaviours; children whose parents had low health literacy often had worse health outcomes; parents with low health literacy had less health knowledge and more behaviours that were less advantageous for their children's health (DeWalt and Hink, 2009).

A range of clear and simple communication strategies have been developed which can be used by nurses and other healthcare professionals to improve health literacy (Dickens and Piano, 2013).

Intentional non-adherence: this type of non-adherence refers to the patient deciding either not to adhere at all, or choosing to follow a treatment regimen in a way different from that recommended, for instance, taking fewer doses or medications, or stopping a course of treatment early.

Of course, a dichotomous model of adherence which defines it as intentional versus unintentional is simplistic. This is recognised by the model's author (Horne, 2006): 'non-adherence related to depression may have both intentional (the patient gives up) and unintentional components (effects on memory and other abilities)', so in any patient there may be overlap of the two concepts. Nevertheless, recognition of the patient as an active decision maker in their treatment adherence has led to research that considers the potentially modifiable factors which motivate people to initiate and persist with treatment regimens (Horne, 2006). The bulk of the evidence is around health beliefs or illness perceptions. Factors associated with medications adherence are illustrated in the case example 'Medications adherence'.

Case Example: Medications adherence

Kirstie is 28 years old and has given up work to look after her six-month-old baby, Georgia, full time. Kirstie and her husband, Rohan, both have asthma for which they have been prescribed a steroid inhaler to be taken regularly (twice a day) and a bronchodilator to be taken as needed. Kirstie's asthma has generally been well controlled. In the past, Rohan's asthma has been troublesome and he has periodically needed short courses of oral steroids.

In the last few months, however, Rohan's asthma has been well controlled. Rohan deliberately changed his routine so that he has developed a habit of taking his steroid inhaler just before he brushes his teeth in the morning and at night. He hardly ever forgets to take it and is feeling the benefit. There is a pharmacy opposite his office so it is easy for him to collect his repeat prescriptions.

Since Georgia's arrival, however, Kirstie has not been taking her inhaler as regularly as she used to. As for most people, having a baby has meant big changes to her routine. Kirstie and Georgia do not have a structure to their day. Kirstie doesn't mind this as she currently has no other responsibilities and is enjoying the break from her daily commute and set office hours; it is hard to fit in errands however. Kirstie has been late collecting her prescription the last couple of times it was due; this has meant she has missed taking her steroid inhaler for several days in a row.

Kirstie is not too worried about missing out on her inhalers as she hasn't noticed any big problems with her breathing yet. She has also noted that not fulfilling her prescription saves a fair bit of money, which she appreciates now that her income is reduced and there are so many new expenses related to Georgia.

 ## Activity: Reflection

Notice how Kirstie's and Rohan's adherence levels have changed over time and with their circumstances. Why might this be? Which elements of their behaviour are intentional and which are non-intentional?

The Role of Illness Perceptions in Non-adherence

There is considerable evidence across a range of conditions that a person's beliefs about their illness, or about its management, predict treatment adherence. Some examples are: belief that coronary artery disease is acute rather than chronic predicted non-adherence to dual antiplatelet therapy (DAPT) (Fennessy et al., 2013); (overly optimistic) belief in graft longevity was related to higher medication non-adherence six months post-kidney transplant (Massey et al., 2013); concern about the benefits of medication was a significant predictor of non-adherence by elderly patients to antihypertensive medication regimens (Rajpura and Nayak, 2014);

adherence was worse in children with asthma whose parents had a more negative perception of the condition, who doubted the necessity for inhaled steroids and who had more concerns about side effects (Morton et al., 2014).

Of course, beliefs around illness and treatments may be entirely rational, for instance when experienced side effects are perceived as worse than the experienced benefits of a treatment. It is when illness or treatment perceptions are based on misconceptions that they are problematic and when healthcare professionals can intervene.

⚙ Activity: Reflection

Consider the likely impact of the following illness perceptions and beliefs about treatments on treatment adherence.

- My diabetes was caused by the pills the doctor gave me for my heart problems
- These asthma inhalers will stunt my child's growth
- I haven't noticed any change in my heart condition since taking the new pills, but I hate they way they make me so sleepy during the day
- My heart disease was caused by stress; smoking makes me less stressed

---

Illness perceptions associated with treatment adherence have been divided by researchers into those which relate to perceptions of the need for treatment and those which relate to concerns about potential adverse consequences. This conceptualisation is known as the 'Necessity–Concerns Framework' (NCF) (Horne and Weinman, 1999). Most of the research is around adherence to prescribed medications. The Beliefs about Medicines Questionnaire has well-validated subscales for measuring necessity beliefs and concerns (Horne et al., 1999). Items such as 'Without my medicines I would become very ill' (necessity belief) and 'I sometimes worry about the long-term effects of my medicines' (concern) are rated on a 5-point Likert scale ranging from 'totally disagree' to 'totally agree'.

The NCF predicts that medication adherence will be associated with stronger perceptions of necessity for treatment and fewer concerns about adverse consequences. This was supported by the findings of a well-conducted systematic review of studies (n=94, participants=25,072) (Horne et al., 2013) of patients with a range of LTCs: asthma, renal disease, organ transplantation, dialysis chronic pain, kidney transplantation, cancer, cardiovascular disorders, Marfan's syndrome, depression, haemophilia, diabetes, HIV, rheumatoid arthritis, osteoporosis, thalassemia, inflammatory bowel disease, bipolar disorder, schizophrenia, epilepsy, migraine, back problems, glaucoma and mixed chronic illness. Meta-analysis indicated that for each standard deviation increase in necessity beliefs, the odds of adherence increased by a factor of 1.7, and for each standard deviation increase in concerns, the odds of adherence decreased by a factor of 2.0.

This work shows that when concerns outweigh necessity beliefs people are likely to be less adherent and vice versa (see Figure 3.1). What happens, however, when people are ambivalent, that is they hold both strong concerns and strong necessity

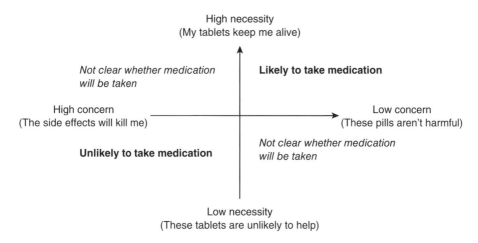

Figure 3.1   The Necessity–Concerns Framework and adherence to medication (see Horne and Weinman, 1999)

Adapted from: Horne et al. (2013) and Clatworthy et al. (2009) with permission from Elsevier

beliefs or when people are indifferent, that is they hold both weak concerns and weak necessity beliefs? Research in stroke survivors (Phillips et al., 2014) (n=600) found that patients with ambivalent attitudes had lower self-reported adherence than patients with indifferent attitudes. In contrast, as noted by Phillips and colleagues (2014) earlier research in blood donors (n=1000) found that more blood was donated by those who were ambivalent compared with those who were indifferent towards blood donation (Gardner and Cacioppo, 1995). Phillips and colleagues (2014) suggest that these conflicting findings warrant further investigation: future research should test whether negative evaluations are generally more predictive of behaviour than positive evaluations, or whether the effects of positive and negative evaluations are illness and/or treatment dependent. Findings would have implications for interventions to change illness or treatment perceptions.

⚙️ Activity: Reflection

Think of examples of necessity beliefs and concerns which may interfere with treatment adherence in your own patients.

Improving Treatment Adherence

A Cochrane review of interventions to improve medication adherence identified 182 RCTs across a range of conditions (Nieuwlaat et al., 2014). The reviewers found that effects were inconsistent across studies, but that even the most effective interventions did not lead to large improvements. The interventions tested were complex and used different approaches. Only five of the identified RCTs improved both medicine adherence and clinical outcomes; the reviewers could not identify any common characteristics for their effectiveness.

Nevertheless, from the discussion above, it would appear that interventions to improve adherence are more likely to be effective if they are tailored to the needs of the individual by taking into account both the person's illness and treatment perceptions and relevant sources of unintentional non-adherence, such as finances, access, cognitive ability and lifestyle. This kind of personalised approach is fundamental to shared decision-making (Horne et al., 2013), which is essential for effective self-management. However, it appears that healthcare professionals, including nurses, often do not ask about patients' illness and treatment perceptions and that consultations may be limited to provision of brief details about medicines and the expected regime (Latter et al., 2010).

This is important since many patients may be reluctant to admit their non-adherence or even to express their concerns about recommended treatments as they may worry about 'offending' their healthcare professional or, perhaps, they may fear less favourable treatment. Nurses, midwives and health visitors therefore need excellent communication skills and a 'no-blame approach' (Horne et al., 2013) if they are to help patients identify and overcome their personal barriers to treatment adherence. With guidance, clinicians can improve their medications-related consultations. A self-efficacy-based framework was used to train nurse prescribers to use an evidence-based intervention to influence exploration of beliefs about medicines in diabetes (Latter et al., 2010); use of the intervention increased patients' initiative in discussion of medicines and increased discussion of concerns about medicines, consequences of non-adherence, attitudes to medication and patient opinions about medicines.

Models for effective consultations have also been developed and applied to promoting treatment adherence. Nurses, midwives and health visitors may be familiar with the Calgary Cambridge model of healthcare consultation (Kurtz et al., 1998, 2003), which was originally developed for medical consultations. Consultation models help clinicians to apply effective communication skills such as active listening, appropriate use of open and closed questions and rapport development in a structured manner, which involves considering each consultation in a series of stages. Stages typically include initiation of the consultation, gathering of information, providing explanations and developing a treatment plan and ending the consultation. Here we consider the Medication-related Consultation Framework (MRCF) (Abdel-Tawab et al., 2011) which has been developed specifically to improve communication around medications.

The MRCF (Abdel-Tawab et al., 2011) is a patient-centred approach which focuses on establishing what is important to the individual patient agenda in respect of their illness and its management. The structured approach to the consultation ensures that both perceptions (intentional factors) and practical problems (unintentional factors) which hinder treatment adherence are identified. Solutions are then developed through a process of shared decision-making. The MRCF considers the consultation in terms of four key phases which are described in Table 3.1.

The MRCF is evidence based in that it was developed through literature review and expert consultation and then refined based on pharmacists' ratings of recorded consultations; psychometric properties of the model were tested during its development and the MRCF was found to discriminate between good, satisfactory and poor consultations (Abdel-Tawab et al., 2011).

Table 3.1 Summary of the Medication-related Consultation Framework

Consultation Phase	Action	Purpose
Scene setting	Introductions; explanation of purpose, scope and structure of consultation.	Establish therapeutic relationship; enable the patient to establish their agenda.
Information gathering	Collect information from the patient about their medicine taking and what they understand about their illness and its treatment; identify barriers to adherence.	Understand the patient's perception of the link between their illness and its treatment; identify the patient's medication-related needs.
Actions and solutions	Identify goals around medication taking; provide risk benefit information.	Agree an acceptable management plan with the patient.
Closing	Agree actions to be taken if the patient experiences difficulties following the treatment plan; assess need for additional information; agree follow-up plan.	Ensure patient safety.

From Abdel-Tawab et al. (2011) with permission from Elsevier

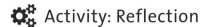 **Activity: Reflection**

The MRCF is not limited to formal consultations, the principles may be applied any time you are discussing a patient's treatment with them. Think back to the last time you had a conversation with a patient about their treatment, consider how your interaction matched the MRCF. How could your interaction have been improved?

Ask yourself: did I introduce myself clearly? Did I find out what concerns the patient had? What were they? What is the patient's explanation for their illness or symptoms? What do they think are the benefits and harms of their treatment regimen? How do these beliefs help or hinder their adherence to their treatment regimen? What needs to be done? Did I end the conversation by making sure that the patient understood what we had discussed and was clear about what to do?

SELF-MANAGEMENT IN A WIDER CONTEXT

This chapter has focused on self-management by patients supported by healthcare professionals; however, the role of systems factors, such as collaboration between multi-disciplinary professionals and between care systems (for instance between primary and secondary care) must also be considered when discussing the management of LTCs, especially in the context of multimorbidity where, due to increased clinical complexity, multi-disciplinary/agency input will be essential.

Examples of approaches to self-management of LTCs which consider whole systems are the 'Chronic Care Model' (Wagner, 1998; Bodenheimer et al., 2002) and 'minimally disruptive medicine' (May et al., 2009).

The Chronic Care Model

The 'Chronic Care Model' (Wagner, 1998; Bodenheimer et al., 2002) was designed to improve LTC management in primary care (from where most people with LTCs receive most care). The model has six components (Stellefson et al., 2013):

- self-management support – facilitating skills-based learning and patient empowerment
- clinical information systems – tracking progress through reporting outcomes to patients and providers
- delivery system redesign – coordinating care processes
- decision support – guidance for implementing evidence-based care
- healthcare organisation – providing leadership for securing resources and removing barriers to care
- community resources and policies – sustaining care by using community-based resources and public health policy

It predicts that these components can produce 'system reform in which informed, activated patients interact with prepared, proactive practice teams' (Kennedy et al., 2013). While the model is intuitive – each of these components appears necessary for effective management of LTCs – the success of the model in different settings has been varied, with some but not all components having been implemented (Bodenheimer et al., 2002). For instance, in the UK, clinical information systems and decision support have been implemented through the Quality and Outcomes Framework (BMA, 2003) which rewards GPs for doing so, but improvements in self-management support have not been incentivised (Kennedy et al., 2013). It would appear that further studies which focus on how best the model can be implemented are needed.

Minimally Disruptive Medicine

The minimally disruptive medicine approach was proposed in response to recognitions of two major problems in the management of LTCs – poor adherence to treatment and uncoordinated and increasing burden on health services. The approach emphasises harmonisation of treatment to reduce the burden on patients, especially in those with multimorbidity, while still pursuing patient goals (May et al., 2009). In the case of mental and physical health co-morbidity, synergistic interventions, such as exercise, **mindfulness** approaches, and social prescribing, which improve both mental and physical health outcomes, are potential minimally disruptive interventions, though 'finding practical and replicable ways of identifying and intervening to take advantage of such synergies' has been identified as a key research and policy priority (Mercer et al., 2012).

CHAPTER SUMMARY

The work involved and skills needed by patients to self-manage long-term conditions in order to reduce morbidity and mortality and to improve quality of life was discussed.

Interventions to support self-management were described; these are most likely to be effective if they are designed to enhance patient self-efficacy.

Self-management support is best provided through shared decision-making which takes into account the individual patient's preferences and goals. Treatment plans are most effective if they are agreed with patients and based on consideration of the patient's perceptions about their illness and its treatment as well as their social circumstances.

A structured approach to consultations can help nurses, midwives and health visitors to understand the patient's beliefs and how these impact on treatment adherence.

Self-management support takes place within the context of a multidisciplinary team and healthcare system.

CONSOLIDATE YOUR LEARNING

 Activity: Quiz

(Answers can be found at the end of this book.)

1. What factors contribute to effective self-management?
2. What health behaviours and outcomes are likely to be affected by a person's illness perceptions?
3. According to the 'Perceptions and Practicalities Model' (Horne, 2006), in what two ways can the factors relating to non-adherence to medication be distinguished?
4. According to the 'Necessity–Concerns Framework' (NCF) (Horne and Weinman, 1999), illness perceptions associated with treatment adherence can be classified as relating to what two factors?

Activity: Reflection

Using health psychology to support self-management

- Think about how you can apply what you have learnt in this chapter to supporting your patients' self-management of their LTC(s)
- What can you do to enhance their self-efficacy?
- What tools could you use to support their self-management?
- How can you find out their illness and treatment perceptions?
- What can you do to help them stick with an agreed plan of care?

FURTHER READING

Multimorbidity: Mercer, S.W., Gunn, J., Bower, P., Wyke, S. and Guthrie, B. (2012) Managing patients with mental and physical multimorbidity. *BMJ*. 345:e5559.
Health coaching: Howard, L.M. and Ceci, C. (2013) Problematizing health coaching for chronic illness self-management. *Nursing Inquiry*. 20(3): 223–31.
Illness perceptions: Marks, D.F., Murray, M., Evans, B. and Estacio, E.V. (2011) Lay representations of illness, in *Health Psychology: Theory, Research and Practice*. (Third edition). London: Sage.

USEFUL WEBSITES

Shared decision-making and decision aids – http://sdm.rightcare.nhs.uk/
Medications consultations – practical resources aimed at pharmacists that are also useful for nurses, midwives and health visitors: Consultation skills for pharmacy practice, NHS Health Education England. http://hee.nhs.uk/work-programmes/pharmacy/consultation-skills-for-pharmacy-practice/

4 PROMOTING HEALTHY CHOICES

Key Learning Objectives

At the end of this chapter you will be able to explain:

- Theoretical approaches to understanding health behaviour change in individuals. These include:

  o Self-determination Theory
  o Temporal Self-regulation Theory
  o The Strength Model of Self-control
  o Relapse prevention

- Psychological constructs involved in health behaviour change in individuals, including:

  o Intention
  o Self-regulation
  o Habit
  o Self-control

- Techniques for helping people to make and stick with healthy choices. These include:

  o Ask, advise, act
  o Feedback and monitoring
  o Goal setting
  o Action planning
  o Coping planning
  o Incentives
  o Motivational interviewing

- Methodological challenges in studying health behaviour change in individuals
- Population-level behaviour change

INTRODUCTION

In spite of a plethora of health education initiatives, many people have difficulty making and sticking to healthy choices. This chapter will focus on understanding why this is the case and will describe behaviour change theories and techniques which nurses, midwives and health visitors can use to help their patients. The information in Chapter 3, especially that concerning self-efficacy and **illness perceptions,** is also relevant to making healthy choices; it will be useful to bear this in mind when reading this chapter.

A substantial cause of population morbidity, mortality and disabling condition impact is strongly related to lifestyle and health behaviours. NICE guidance (2014a) on individual-level behaviour change interventions for people aged 16 and over identifies helping patients to improve diet, increase exercise, stop smoking, reduce alcohol intake and to practise safe sex as important for long-term health and quality of life. Nurses, midwives and health visitors have a key role in helping their patients to make and to stick to healthy choices around these and other illness prevention behaviours such as attending for cancer screening, diabetic retinopathy screening, periodic health checks for long-term conditions or for annual physical health checks for people diagnosed with a severe mental illness. The final section of this chapter will put individual behaviour change in context by briefly discussing public health or population-level behaviour change interventions.

BEHAVIOUR CHANGE – INDIVIDUAL LEVEL

Individual-level behaviour change interventions are designed to cause measureable change within an individual. They may be opportunistic or planned. They vary in intensity from single interventions to high-intensity interventions or therapies which may involve a course of sessions. They may be delivered one-to-one or in groups, in person or remotely (for example by telephone or via the internet).

The ability to change or modify one's behaviour is termed 'self-regulation' (see Box 4.1: Self-regulation). A range of self-regulatory behaviours and techniques to promote and sustain these behaviours have been defined and tested in research. In order to help you to critically appraise this research, some of the methodological issues involved are discussed next.

Box 4.1: Self-regulation

- Self-regulation is the ability to change, alter or modify one's own behaviour (Hagger, 2010) often in the pursuit of a specific goal (Carver and Scheier, 1998)
- Self-regulatory behaviours are actions that have the expressed purpose of changing or modifying behaviour (Sniehotta et al., 2005; Hagger, 2010)
- Self-regulatory behaviours are conscious, intentional and goal directed (rather than habitual or unconscious) and require effort and planning (Sniehotta et al., 2005; Hagger et al., 2010)

- Constructs such as intentions, **motivation**, self-efficacy, perceived control, **attitudes** and beliefs as specified by **health psychology models** and theories are correlated with self-regulation (Hagger, 2010).
- Evidence-based health behaviour change techniques which target self-regulation commonly involve setting goals and planning how to achieve them (action planning), including how to overcome difficulties (coping planning).
- Monitoring of and regular feedback on progress help sustain self-regulatory behaviours.

BEHAVIOUR CHANGE – RESEARCH

Despite increased understanding of behaviour change processes and the development of behaviour change interventions, rising rates of conditions related to unhealthy lifestyles, such as diabetes (Wild et al., 2004), suggest that there remains much to learn. Some methodological challenges of behaviour change research have been identified and will need to be overcome in order to improve knowledge.

Theories of Behaviour Change

Health psychology theories provide a framework for understanding the cognitive, behavioural, attitudinal and environmental factors which influence making and maintaining healthy choices. Theories such as the Health Belief Model (Rosenstock, 1966; Becker, 1974), Stages of Change Model (Prochaska and DiClemente, 1983; Prochaska et al., 1992) and the Theory of Planned Behaviour/Reasoned Action (Fishbein and Ajzen, 1975) were discussed in Chapter 1. These help predict health behaviour, but no theory currently captures all the intrinsic and extrinsic factors linked with behaviour change. Furthermore, behaviour change interventions are commonly designed without reference to theory or commonly only address some aspects of a theory (Michie et al., 2011b). This makes it difficult to understand how an intervention works.

Michie and colleagues (2011b) have proposed an alternative framework to characterise, choose and design behaviour change interventions – the 'Behaviour Change Wheel'. At the centre of this framework is a behaviour system known as 'COM-B' (see Figure 4.1). C is for 'capability' – the individual's psychological and physical capacity including knowledge and skills, for instance knowing what services are available and understanding the risks of the behaviour; O is for 'opportunity' – the extrinsic environmental and social factors which facilitate or hinder behaviour change, such as cost, available facilities and **social support**; M is for 'motivation' – the reflective (for example decision-making) and automatic (for example habits) determinants of behaviour.

The COM-B model guides assessment of a behaviour to help understand what kind of intervention may be needed to change it. Michie and colleagues (2011b) have also identified processes or 'intervention functions' (e.g. modelling, training, education), which can address deficits in one or more of the COM-B factors. They have also

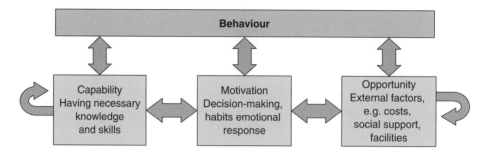

Figure 4.1   The COM-B model for understanding behaviour (Michie et al., 2011b)

defined categories of policy (e.g. guidelines, planning, service provision) that could enable those interventions to occur. As a relatively new development within health psychology, there is as yet limited research that has applied this model.

Reporting of Behaviour Change Interventions

There is a considerable body of research describing the development and evaluation of behaviour change interventions. However, in common with other types of complex interventions (see Box 4.2: Reporting standards for complex interventions), they are often poorly described in studies. This means that it can be difficult for healthcare professionals to apply a new intervention in their clinical practice. In an attempt to address this, a **Delphi-type study** was conducted to develop a taxonomy of behaviour change techniques (Michie et al., 2013). As many as 93 distinct techniques were identified and agreed as a method for specifying behaviour change interventions. Some of the more practical and best-researched techniques are discussed later in this chapter.

Box 4.2: Reporting standards for complex interventions

- Adequate descriptions of interventions are necessary for researchers to replicate or build on research findings and for implementation across settings
- The Consolidated Standards of Reporting Trials (CONSORT) 2010 statement is a guide for authors as to how to report clinical trials, and the standard to which most journal editors expect authors to adhere
- CONSORT states that the interventions for each group within a trial should be reported with 'sufficient details to allow replication, including how and when they were actually administered'
- Despite this guidance, the quality of descriptions of interventions and of their comparisons has been found to be remarkably poor (Hoffman et al., 2014)
- The 'template for intervention description and replication' (TIDieR) checklist and guide (Hoffman et al., 2014) builds on CONSORT to improve reporting of interventions in trials and other evaluation studies

Measuring Behaviour Change

Choosing outcome measures for studies of behaviour change can be difficult. The outcome of interest depends on the target behaviour or on the condition that the behaviour is thought to influence. Objective measures such as biomarkers (for example HbA1c in diabetes or breath carbon monoxide in smoking cessation) may be favoured, but trials may not be of sufficient duration to determine long-term health benefits. Objective measures of behaviours such as appointment keeping, exercise class attendance or medication taking may be used. However, these are only a proxy measure for actual outcome as attendance at pulmonary rehabilitation classes, for instance, may be necessary for improved breathlessness, but not sufficient – other factors such as effort put in, extent of lung damage, skill of the physiotherapist and so on will also impact on whether breathlessness improves.

Subjective measures of behaviour change such as questionnaires, global questions or diaries can be used, but few validated measures exist and different types of measure may obtain different results. In a trial of a primary care behaviour change intervention for smoking, alcohol use, diet and physical activity (Butler et al., 2013), self-reported change at three months differed from that indicated by questionnaire scores. Questionnaires may be less prone to reporting bias but, as the authors note (Butler et al., 2013), perceptions of having made a lasting change and scores from questionnaires may be measuring different constructs.

The intervention in that trial (Butler et al., 2013), which involved training primary care clinicians in behaviour change counselling using a brief blended learning programme, did not improve either self-reported behaviour change or biomedical measures (hip to waist ratio, **body mass index**, cholesterol, blood pressure) at 12 months, but it did increase patients' intentions to change (Butler et al., 2013). Intention to change has been found in a systematic review of 76 studies (Webb and Sheeran, 2006) to predict actual change, at least to some extent: meta-analysis showed that a medium-to-large change in intention (effect size $d = 0.66$) leads to a small-to-medium change in behaviour (effect size $d = 0.36$).

The 12-month duration of the Butler et al. (2013) trial was unusual. A review of behaviour change research used to inform NICE guidance (NICE, 2014a), found that the effectiveness of behaviour change interventions is rarely assessed beyond six to 12 weeks post intervention; this is often due to lack of funding for research studies.

Impact of Clinician Behaviour

The extent to which clinicians are trained in behaviour change techniques, their level of interest and their fidelity to the intervention (see Box 4.3: **Intervention fidelity**) are all likely to affect the impact of behaviour change interventions. Training is important in encouraging clinicians to address lifestyle changes with their patients. Without training, some clinicians have reported lack of confidence in counselling patients on behaviours that they struggle with themselves (Vickers et al., 2007). Unfortunately, a lack of evidence concerning the relationship between practitioner training, subsequent competencies and behaviour change has been identified (NICE, 2014a), so it is unclear how much training and which competencies are needed by clinicians to deliver behaviour change interventions effectively.

Box 4.3: Intervention fidelity

- Defined as 'The degree to which the planned components of an intervention have been delivered as intended' (NICE, 2014a)
- Synonyms include: treatment fidelity, implementation fidelity, program fidelity, treatment integrity and procedural reliability
- Is a **mediator** of study outcomes (Perepletchikova and Kazdin, 2005); a potentially effective intervention may fail to effect change if it is not delivered appropriately.
- Is essential if a study intervention is to be replicated across settings
- May be affected by clinician *adherence* – 'the extent to which a person delivers the essential content, delivery strategies and theories prescribed by the intervention designers and avoids activities proscribed by them', or *competence* – 'the level of "skill" ... may include the ability to respond appropriately to a wide variety of contextual cues' (Mars et al., 2013: 2). The latter being less well defined and measured (Mars et al., 2013: 2)
- May be measured by rating of actual or audio/video recordings of interactions between clinicians and patients or by self-report checklists completed by clinicians to indicate which elements of the intervention they delivered
- Is often inadequately addressed due to a lack of standardised definitions and valid and reliable measures (Cross and West, 2011)

Single Versus Multiple Behaviour Change

There is evidence for the effectiveness of a range of interventions for changing single behaviours (for example, smoking, drinking too much alcohol, and being physically inactive); however, the best approach for addressing multiple unhealthy behaviours (for instance, if someone had all three of those behaviours) is unclear (NICE, 2014a). Research is needed to determine whether more than one behaviour can be tackled effectively simultaneously or whether behaviours should be prioritised for change. If the latter, how – the most damaging (if that can be determined) or the one the patient most wants to change? Furthermore, interventions may be effective for one aspect of behaviour change, but not another, and there is a lack of validated tools for measuring more than one type of behaviour change simultaneously (Butler et al., 2013).

BEHAVIOUR CHANGE – APPLICATION IN CLINICAL PRACTICE

Every healthcare professional should use every contact with an individual to help them maintain or improve their mental and physical health and wellbeing; in particular targeting the four main lifestyle risk factors; diet, physical activity, alcohol and tobacco – whatever their speciality or the purpose of the contact. (NHS, 2012)

Similarly, The Royal College of Nursing (RCN) states that 'every interaction in every location should be seen as an opportunity to promote health and prevent illness'

(RCN, 2012a). This approach is called 'Making Every Contact Count' (MECC) and is a recommendation for every healthcare organisation (NHS, 2012). Guidance and toolkits are available to help (see Further Reading below).

NICE (2014a) guidance distinguishes between '**very brief interventions**', which may take only a few seconds and consist of providing information, or directing people where to get help, and '**brief interventions**', which take a few minutes and may involve discussion, negotiation or encouragement, provision of supportive materials (e.g. information leaflets) and referral for further support. The effectiveness of such interventions is supported by research evidence. For instance, a well-conducted systematic review of 13 RCTs (Aveyard et al., 2012) found that opportunistic brief physician advice to stop smoking on medical grounds and offer of assistance increased the frequency of quit attempts (risk ratio 1.24, 95 per cent confidence interval 1.16–1.33) compared with no intervention.

A Cochrane review (n=49 studies) (Rice et al., 2013) found that nursing or health visitor-delivered interventions for smoking cessation increased the likelihood of quitting compared with usual care. It also found that the effect size from studies (n=7 studies) which used a particularly low intensity intervention was similar to the overall effect size (relative risk 1.29, 95 per cent confidence interval 1.20 to 1.39), although the confidence interval was wider. This indicates that although higher intensity interventions may be more effective, providing simple brief advice is nevertheless beneficial and supports the principle of MECC.

Brief interventions can be delivered by non-specialists with minimal training, are aimed at early intervention and usually delivered to individuals who are not actively seeking treatment (McQueen et al., 2011) (see Box 4.4: The role of intention in behaviour change). A Cochrane review of 14 RCTs (McQueen et al., 2011) of brief interventions delivered to heavy alcohol users who had been admitted to general inpatient hospital care for reasons other than for alcohol treatment exemplifies this. It found that patients receiving brief interventions (between 1 and 3 sessions of 15 to 60 minutes) had a greater reduction in alcohol consumption at six months (mean difference –69.43, 95 per cent confidence interval –128.14 to –10.72) and nine months (mean difference –182.88, 95 per cent confidence interval –360.00 to –5.76) follow up compared with those receiving no or usual care.

Box 4.4: The role of intention in behaviour change

- Intentions are viewed as predictors of behaviour and are at the heart of health psychology theories (see Chapter 1):

  o Intentions are developed following evaluation of a behaviour and its expected consequences, with evaluations mediated by **subjective norms** or social pressures (Theory of Planned Behaviour (Ajzen, 1985, 1991; Ajzen, and Madden 1986) and Reasoned Action (Fishbein and Ajzen, 1975))

  o Intentions are formed following appraisal of threat (severity of outcome, susceptibility to outcome, fear of outcome) and coping (response effectiveness and costs,

(Continued)

(Continued)

self-efficacy) (Protection-motivation Theory (Rogers 1975, 1983), an extension of the Health Belief Model (Rosenstock, 1966; Becker, 1974))

- Evidence from prospective studies shows that intentions predict actual behaviour change at least to some extent (Webb and Sheeran, 2006)
- But many people who intend to change their behaviour are unsuccessful – this is known as the 'intention–behaviour gap' (Sheeran, 2002)
- Behaviour change interventions can facilitate turning intentions into behaviour
- Evidence from studies of opportunistic behaviour change interventions suggests that behaviour change support can be effective even when the patient has not been seeking it

Brief interventions may or may not be structured. An example of a structured approach is the 'ask, advise, act' model. In smoking cessation, this approach's (detailed below as a case example) development has been informed by a review of brief interventions for smoking cessation (Aveyard et al., 2012) and behaviour change competencies (Michie et al., 2011a). Next we will look at some other, more complex, behaviour change techniques, which we as nurses, midwives and health visitors can use to help patients to make healthy choices.

 ## Case Example: Using the 'ask, advise, act' model for smoking cessation

Dinesh is 65 years old, has mild COPD and has an appointment with his practice nurse to receive his annual flu vaccination. The appointment is scheduled to last 5 minutes.

Assess current and past smoking behaviour [ask]

'How many cigarettes do you smoke in a day?'

'Have you tried to stop smoking before?'

(purpose – information gathering)

Provide information on consequences of smoking and smoking cessation [advise]

'You know that smoking will make your bronchitis worse and put you at risk of developing lung cancer?'

'If you stop now, you will notice an improvement in your breathing within months.'

(purpose – focus on behaviour and address motivation)

Provide options for later/additional support [act]

'If you like you can make another appointment to see me and I can provide more support to help you quit; the local pharmacist can also help.'

'You may find the NHS Choices website helpful: www.nhs.uk/livewell/smoking/Pages/stopsmokingnewhome.aspx'

(purpose – encourage action)

Advise on stop smoking medications [act]

'You are more likely to succeed in quitting if you use nicotine replacement patches, electronic cigarettes or medications; I or your GP or the pharmacist can give you more advice about these options.'

(purpose – encourage action)

Note: Evidence suggests that this intervention can be effective whether or not Dinesh suggests that he is ready to quit (Aveyard et al., 2012).

BEHAVIOUR CHANGE TECHNIQUES

The NICE guidance on individual-level behaviour change (NICE, 2014a) was informed by Michie et al.'s (2013) taxonomy of 93 behaviour change techniques. The guideline development group suggests that two groups of techniques – feedback and monitoring and goals and planning – are likely to be effective within interventions to change behaviours relating to alcohol, diet, physical activity and smoking. Techniques utilising social support were also considered potentially helpful. For instance, in one study (Wing and Jeffrey, 1999), people attending a weight loss intervention with friends had a 33 per cent greater weight loss and lower drop out rate at ten months follow up compared with those who attended alone. However, negative effects of social support such as unhealthy co-dependency, bullying and manipulation were also identified by the guideline development group. Therefore behaviour change techniques relating only to feedback and monitoring and to goals and planning are discussed here.

Feedback and Monitoring

Feedback and monitoring involves individuals recording either a behaviour, for instance, number of cigarettes smoked, sugary foods eaten, miles walked in a day, or an outcome, for instance, lung function or weight loss. Records of changes in the behaviour or outcome constitute feedback. Feedback and monitoring can be provided by a healthcare professional (or someone else such as a carer) or by the individual themselves (self-monitoring). Diaries, charts or questionnaire scores can be used to record behaviour and monitor progress.

Records make behaviour explicit, which is important because people's beliefs about what they do often differ from what they actually do (Michie et al., 2008). For instance, someone (motivated by denial, guilt or stigma) may tell themselves that they do not over eat, but a daily food diary shows them how many calories they have actually consumed. Even if their diary entries are not entirely honest (due to **social desirability bias**), the process of making them will increase their self-awareness of their behaviour.

Feedback and monitoring helps individuals to:

- Clarify which behaviours they should target. For instance, recording their eating activity in a daily diary can help an individual to see of what kinds of foods they eat too much
- Make action or coping plans (see below). For instance, a daily food diary may reveal that someone commonly eats sugary snacks in the early evening. Noticing that this is a regular pattern can help them to plan healthier behaviours at this time such as eating fruit, drinking water or doing some kind of activity to distract from cravings
- Modify action or coping plans. Feedback of failures and successes of planned actions can help the individual to understand what is helpful and what is not. For instance, their plan to eat fruit in the early evening may not have been successful, so they decide to go for a walk instead
- Stay motivated. Noticing achievements (mastery experiences, see Chapter 3) increases self-efficacy (Bandura, 1977)

The following goals and planning techniques can be used to structure and guide feedback and monitoring activity.

Goals and Planning

Setting goals and then making a specific plan to achieve those goals allows patients to make small but meaningful behaviour changes (e.g. increasing exercise, reducing alchol intake), which will lead to long-term change (e.g. improved overall health) (Lorig et al., 2014).

Goals

Goals are likely to work as a behaviour change tool via improvement of self-efficacy (Bodenheimer and Handley, 2009; Barley et al., 2014). Goal achievement provides a **mastery experience** which encourages the person to continue with the behaviour or to set a higher goal. Conversely, failure to achieve a goal can reduce feelings of self-efficacy so nurses, midwives and health visitors should guide patients to set goals which are achievable. To ensure this, goals should be 'SMART' – an acronym for 'specific (exactly what will be achieved), measurable (how to know if it has been achieved), achievable (realistic taking into account skills, resources and context), relevant (important to the person), time-bound (when the goal will be accomplished)' (see Box 4.5: SMART goals).

Should your patient fail to achieve their goal, damage to self-efficacy may be limited by you, the healthcare provider, taking joint responsibility for having chosen a goal that was too hard. The reasons why the patient did not achieve the goal can then be explored and a more realistic goal set (Michie et al., 2008).

Box 4.5: SMART goals

	Examples
Specific	General: *I must eat more healthily.* Specific: *I will eat fruit instead of biscuits between meals.*
Measurable	Hard to measure: *I will be more active.* Easy to measure: *I will walk in the park for 20 minutes every Monday, Wednesday and Friday before 11 am.*
Achievable	Difficult to achieve: *I will only eat healthy food from now on.* Easier to achieve: *I will eat five portions of fruit or vegetables each day this week.*
Relevant	Not relevant: *I will stop smoking because the nurse says I should.* Relevant: *I will stop smoking because I am fed up with coughing when I wake up each morning.*
Time-bound	No time frame: *I will lose weight.* With time frame: *I will achieve my target weight within six months.*

For any patient, the target of the chosen goal may either be selected by a health professional or by the patient themselves. In research, the former approach is typically taken as trials are designed around a particular behaviour such as increasing physical exercise or alcohol intake. These may also reflect targets in your clinical area. Personalised goal-setting, where the patient selects which behaviour to target, has also been tested (Barley et al., 2014) but it can be difficult to select an outcome measure which captures changes in patients who are addressing unrelated behaviours and therefore difficult to determine the effectiveness of this approach. In either case the details of the SMART goal (and plan, see below) should be personalised or tailored to the individual because this makes them more likely to be responsive to the patient's needs and to lead to better outcomes (Liddell et al., 2008; Elwell et al., 2013; NICE, 2014a).

Action Planning and Coping Planning

Goal attainment is more likely if an individual has an action plan which specifies when, where and how to perform a behaviour. Action planning has been shown to be beneficial for a range of health-related behaviours including smoking cessation, healthy eating, exercising, oral hygiene, breast self-examination, stair use and taking vitamin supplements (Kwasnicka et al., 2013). Furthermore, a systematic review of 11 RCTs and quasi-RCTs (Kwasnicka et al., 2013) suggests that additional inclusion of a 'coping plan' which specifies how to deal with anticipated barriers to achieving a desired behaviour will be even more effective. Action planning and coping planning are also important for relapse prevention (see Box 4.6: Relapse prevention).

Box 4.6: Relapse prevention

Many people may be able to make a healthy change in the short term, but later return to their old ways (relapse).

The most well-known model of relapse prevention is Marlatt and Gordon's (1985) cognitive behavioural model of relapse prevention.

The model predicts that, in a high-risk situation, effective coping will lead to increased self-efficacy and a lower probability of relapse.

Relapse prevention interventions include identifying high-risk situations for an individual and enhancing their coping by providing psychoeducation, addressing unhelpful beliefs and using behaviour change techniques to increase their self-efficacy.

Relapse prevention interventions have been studied mostly with regard to alcohol and drug use and other addictive behaviours (Hendershot et al., 2011), including smoking cessation (Hajek et al., 2013), but can be applied to any kind of long-term behaviour change.

Patients should be encouraged to record their goals and plans for achieving them in writing; this is likely to increase their perceived control, which is a correlate of behaviour change (Andersson and Conley, 2008). Free worksheets for goal setting and action planning can be found easily online. Interventions which nurses, midwives and health visitors can use to help with action planning and coping planning include: identifying barriers and facilitators, **implementation intentions** and **behavioural contracts**.

Identifying barriers and facilitators: Once a barrier has been identified, an individual can develop a realistic view of its likely impact and can be helped to develop strategies for overcoming it: a technique known as 'problem solving'. A specific coping plan can then be devised. From your clinical experience, you may already have some idea of what factors can prevent patients from making and enacting healthy choices, but, in order to ensure that coping plans are personalised and achievable, it is also important to ask the patient what they think may get in the way. Similarly, asking patients what may help them to achieve their goal is important: past successful strategies for achieving similar goals or which helped overcome similar barriers (facilitators) can then be applied in the new situation. The case example below highlights some barriers and facilitators for attending cancer screening.

Case Example: Barriers and facilitators for attending for a cervical cancer screening appointment

Jeong-Su is 27 years old. During her annual asthma check, her practice nurse notices that she has not attended for her routine cervical cancer screen. The nurse asks if she would like to book an appointment. Jeong-Su seems unsure, so the nurse asks her what is wrong. They identify the following potential barriers:

- Lack of understanding of what the test is for and what it involves
- Fear that the test will hurt
- Difficulty taking time off work to attend healthcare appointments additional to her asthma checks

Between them, Jeong-Su and the nurse agree what could help (facilitators):

- The nurse explains the procedure in detail, including showing Jeong-Su the speculum which will be used
- A leaflet explaining the risk and benefits of attending is provided
- The nurse encourages Jeong-Su to talk to friends and family about their experience (if Jeong-Su can identify specific individuals she will be more likely to do this)
- The nurse explains to Jeong-Su which days the surgery is open late and that she could also attend her local well woman clinic one evening to get the test (address and opening times provided)

Jeong-Su is reassured a little, but wants to think it over. She and the nurse agree that she will ring the surgery by the end of the week if she wants to have the test. (This simple action plan will make it more likely that Jeong-Su will think things over and make a decision, rather than postponing indefinitely.)

One approach to identifying barriers and facilitators is to ask patients how confident they are that they can achieve their goal (Michie et al., 2008); use of a '**confidence ruler**' – a scale from 1 (not at all) to 10 (extremely confident) can help to focus the conversation. Once an individual has specified a number, the health professional can either ask 'what would help to make that higher?' or, if it is already high, ask them why – this enables them to make their facilitators explicit so that they are more available mentally and easier to draw on in the face of a barrier. If the patient's confidence is very low, it may be best to start with a more achievable goal. Achievement of an easier goal should increase self-efficacy for more complex, subsequent goals.

Remember that barriers and facilitators may be internal (for example, emotional responses, level of knowledge, beliefs) or external (for example, cost, access, availability of social support).

> ## ⚙ Activity: Reflection
>
> Re-read the section on Treatment Adherence in Chapter 3. Consider how this applies to adhering to healthy choices. In particular, consider the kinds of beliefs or perceptions which may help or hinder. For instance, believing that 'only gay men catch HIV' may lead to not using condoms; believing that 'physically fit people live longer' may lead to exercising more. Unhelpful beliefs can be challenged through discussion of the research evidence.
>
>   Identify a goal for healthy living for someone typical of one of your patients. What kind of barriers might they experience for achieving it? What facilitators might they have, or could you provide?

Implementation intentions: Also known as 'conditional plans' or 'if–then rules', implementation intentions are proposed as an internal memory strategy to instigate goal-directed behaviour in the presence of a contextual cue (Gollwitzer and Brandstatter, 1997). Implementation intentions take the form of **If** 'x' happens/situation arises, **then** I will execute behaviour 'y'. For example: 'If it is a Monday morning, **then** I will go for a walk in the park', or '**If** I feel like a cigarette, **then** I will suck a sweet instead'. Systematic reviews of RCT evidence support the effectiveness of implemention intentions in goal attainment across multiple behaviours (Gollwitzer and Sheeran, 2006) including healthy eating (Adriaanse et al., 2011) and physical activity (Belanger-Gravel et al., 2011).

A variety of mechanisms through which the formulation of implementation intentions is thought to help behaviour change have been proposed. Implementation intentions improve planning capacity, help people to notice opportunities to act before it is too late, act as a trigger or reminder for positive behaviour, link barriers with facilitators and help to develop new good habits (see Box 4.7: The role of habit in behaviour change) so that the positive behaviour becomes automatic (Michie et al., 2008; Gollwitzer and Sheeran, 2006), reducing the need for **self-control** (see below).

Box 4.7: The role of habit in behaviour change

Habits are actions (for example, washing hands) that are triggered automatically in response to contextual cues (for example, after touching a patient) (Gardner et al., 2012).

    Habits can be adaptive as their automaticity frees mental resources for other tasks.

    When behaviour is habitual, intentions are poor predictors of behaviour (Van't Riet et al., 2011).

    It is not possible to form a habit for not doing something, so patients should be advised to choose a new behaviour in order to form a new healthy habit (Gardner et al., 2012) – for example, eating fruit at breakfast.

It is much harder to break a habit than make a new one, therefore consider advising patients to replace an old habit with a new one – for example, eat sweets or play with keys instead of reaching for a cigarette.

Based on daily repetition, patients should be advised that it may take around 10 weeks to form a new habit (Gardner et al., 2012).

Behavioural contracts: In healthcare, behavioural contracts are verbal or written agreements between a healthcare professional and a patient which provide a record of what goals and actions have been agreed. If a reward is attached to completing the specified actions, this is known as a 'contingency contract' – the reward is contingent on fulfilment of the contract. Making a contract is seen as a sign of the commitment of the two parties to adhere to the agreed plan. A Cochrane review (Bosch-Capblanch et al., 2007) of the effects of contracts between patients and healthcare practitioners for improving patients' adherence to treatment, prevention and health promotion activities found 30 RCTs (n=4691) comparing contracts associated with a range of behaviours (including addictions and weight loss) with usual care or another active intervention. About half of the trials found a favourable effect compared with the control condition in at least one outcome. This suggests that it may be worth considering using contracts in clinical practice; however, most of the trials were of poor quality, so the authors conclude that the evidence base is insufficient to recommend their routine use.

The behaviour change approaches described above are largely informed by cognitive or behavioural theories in which outcomes depend on how we think and/or how we act. For instance, we will be more likely to reduce our alcohol intake if we think doing so is important (**cognition**) and we will exercise more if make a plan (behaviour) to do so. Lay people, however, commonly focus on the importance of 'will power' or 'self-control' in regulating their behaviour; we discuss this next.

SELF-CONTROL

Self-control refers to an individual's ability to override their learned behaviours or habits. The Strength Model of Self-control (Muraven and Baumeister, 2000; Baumeister et al., 2007) has been proposed to explain how self-control underpins an individual's capacity to engage in self-regulatory behaviours, including health behaviours.

The Strength Model of Self-control (Muraven and Baumeister, 2000; Baumeister et al., 2007)

This proposes that self-control is like a muscle – if we over-exert our self-control 'muscle' it becomes fatigued and less effective. In an experiment to test this, participants forced to resist the temptation to eat treats by eating healthy radishes instead subsequently gave up trying to solve an unsolvable puzzle faster than people who had not previously exerted self-control (Baumeister et al., 1998). This and other similar experiments indicate that self-control is a limited resource. Many behaviours, such as consuming too much alcohol or sugary foods and resting instead of being active, are tempting because they are pleasurable in the short term; the strength model explains why relying on self-control to resist temptation is unlikely to work – the more we use our self-control the quicker it runs out! Hence it is more effective to keep out of temptation's way (don't buy those biscuits!), than it is to actively resist it (ignore the biscuits in the cupboard).

There is nevertheless some evidence that an individual's capacity for self-control can be increased. As is the case with other muscles, regular exercise (avoiding over exertion) may strengthen the self-control 'muscle'. Baumeister et al. (2006) reviewed experimental studies designed to increase self-control in a range of behaviours and found that exercising self-control for one behaviour increased self-control for other very different behaviours. For example, study participants who had adhered to a regular exercise programme for two months (i.e. had exercised their self-control for resisting inactivity) showed greater overall self-control compared with controls; this was evidenced by greater success in reducing cigarette smoking, alcohol use, caffeine and junk food consumption and impulsive spending, and by eating more healthy food, studying more, watching less television as well as by their reported greater emotional control (Oaten and Cheng, 2006). Insufficient research has been conducted to determine whether including self-control strengthening exercises in behaviour change interventions is beneficial however (Hagger et al., 2010).

So, thoughts, behaviours and personality appear to be important for behaviour change. The concept of 'motivation' has also been considered. Self-determination Theory (Deci and Ryan, 1985) has been proposed to explain the role of 'intrinsic motivation' in behaviour change. Intrinsic motivation comes from within, as opposed to 'extrinsic motivation', which is linked to rewards and incentives, which are discussed further below.

SELF-DETERMINATION THEORY (SDT) (DECI AND RYAN, 1985)

This proposes that individuals are more likely to participate and persist in behaviours that they find enjoyable or which reflect their **values** than in behaviours which are externally driven; for instance, through reward or avoidance of punishment. Intrinsically driven behaviours satisfy a basic psychological need for '**autonomy**'. This is the need of an individual to feel that they are responsible for and have chosen their actions. Two additional basic psychological needs are also proposed to be important: 'competence' (the need to feel effective) and 'relatedness' (the need to feel understood and cared for by others) (Ng et al., 2012). Greater fulfilment of these needs has been found to be associated with better mental and physical health and more healthy behaviour (Ng et al., 2012).

SDT predicts that a patient's level of autonomy, competence and relatedness will be increased in healthcare contexts which are 'autonomy-supportive', that is contexts where patient perspectives and choices are considered. This was supported by a meta-analytic review (Ng et al., 2012) of 184 studies that applied SDT to health behaviours such as physical activity, diabetes care, abstinence from tobacco, and weight control. Behaviour change interventions informed by SDT therefore aim to help individuals to internalise and value healthy behaviours. See Box 4.8 for an example of an SDT-informed intervention.

Box 4.8: A weight management intervention based on SDT (Silva et al., 2010)

An RCT (n=239 women) was conducted which tested the effectiveness of an SDT-informed intervention compared with an educational intervention in increasing physical activity and reducing weight.

At 12 months, the women in the SDT group showed greater weight loss (−7.29 per cent) and higher levels of physical activity/exercise (+138 ± 26 min/day of moderate plus vigorous exercise; +2,049 ± 571 steps/day) compared to those in the control group (p < 0.001).

The intervention was designed to create an autonomy-supportive environment, which promoted in each participant 'a sense of ownership over their behaviour such that it would stem from an internal perceived locus of causality'.

This involved (reported in Silva et al., 2010):

1. building sustainable knowledge that supported informed choices, by using neutral language during interpersonal communication (e.g. 'may' and 'could', and not 'should' or 'must').
2. encouraging choice and self-initiation; the use of prescriptions, pressure, demands and extrinsic rewards were minimal if not absent.
3. providing participants with a menu of options and a variety of avenues for behaviour change.
4. supporting the presentation of tasks and choices with a clear rationale to adopt a specific behaviour by presenting clear contingencies between behaviour and outcome.
5. encouraging participants to build and explore congruence between their values and goals, and their lifestyles.
6. giving informational positive feedback, acknowledging that the feeling of competence grows from feedback inherent to the task (cues for objective success).

Although interventions informed by SDT appear to have potential for promoting health behaviour change, to date few SDT interventions have been developed and tested. SDT has been proposed (Markland et al., 2005; Miller and Rollnick, 2012a), however, as a conceptual framework for a very well-tested behaviour change intervention – 'Motivational Interviewing' (MI; Miller and Rollnick, 1991), which we will discuss next.

MOTIVATIONAL INTERVIEWING (MI) (MILLER AND ROLLNICK, 1991)

MI is 'a collaborative, goal-oriented style of communication which pays particular attention to the language of change. It is designed to strengthen personal motivation for and commitment to a specific goal by eliciting and exploring the person's own reasons for change within an atmosphere of acceptance and compassion' (Miller and Rollnick, 2012b: 29). The key concepts within MI and the skills that clinicians need to implement them are detailed in Box 4.9.

Box 4.9: Motivational Interviewing: key concepts and skills

Key concepts: the aim of MI is to shape a conversation so that the patient talks themselves into making a change that will be beneficial to them. It involves:

Collaboration – a process of negotiation rather than persuasion or confrontation, which are likely to produce **resistance** to change. Clinicians should 'roll with resistance' – instead of challenging the person, they should help them to explore their reasons for their resistance.

Eliciting the person's own reasons for change – patients are encouraged to talk about why they want to change to reveal their intrinsic motivation. Advice or information is only provided if the person requests it.

Acceptance – being non-judgemental and respecting the person's wishes, even if they decide not to make a change: this supports the patient's autonomy.

Compassion – showing empathy, concern for the person's welfare and acknowledging their efforts and struggles.

Key skills: The acronym 'OARS' can help you to remember four key skills used in MI.

Open-ended questions – encourage the patient to do most of the talking.

Affirmation – be supportive; make positive or complimentary comments about the person's strengths, abilities and efforts.

Reflective listening – pay attention to the person, do not judge or interrupt, allow for silences; focus on their change talk.

Summarising – repeat to the person what they have been telling you. This demonstrates empathy and builds rapport. Salient points can be highlighted to shift the direction of the conversation towards change.

MI was first developed to treat alcohol problems, but has since been used and found effective for a range of lifestyle problems and in improving self-management of LTCs.

A systematic review of 48 RCTs (9,618 participants) of MI in medical settings found benefit for a range of outcomes including: HIV viral load, dental outcomes, death rate, body weight, alcohol and tobacco use, sedentary behaviour, self-monitoring, confidence in change, and approach to treatment (Lundahl et al., 2013). MI is an intuitive approach developed from clinical experience rather than any particular theory of behaviour change (Miller and Rollnick, 2012a). Researchers have nevertheless tried to understand the processes through which MI is effective and there is some evidence that the three psychological needs underpinning Self-determination Theory (autonomy, relatedness, and competence) are all directly addressed in MI (Markland et al., 2005; Miller and Rollnick, 2012a).

MI has been recommended by the Royal College of Nursing (RCN, 2015) as an excellent tool for using with MECC across the community, 'from discussing medication with a client and why they are reluctant to take certain drugs, or talking to a family about keeping children off school to prevent cross infection or even supporting a client who is anxious or depressed'.

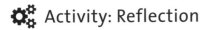 **Activity: Reflection**

Think about how you usually talk with patients or their carers about making healthy choices. Do you give them advice or try to persuade them to change? How well does that work? Next time you meet a patient who is resisting healthy choices, try applying the motivational interviewing approach. See what happens – did it change your relationship with them? Did they seem less resistant in the end?

The theories and techniques considered so far account for behaviour change mainly in terms of internal processes, however, our environment is also likely to have an impact. The following Temporal Self-regulation Theory (Hall and Fong, 2007) has been proposed to account for this and is considered next.

TEMPORAL SELF-REGULATION THEORY (TST) (HALL AND FONG, 2007)

As we know, unhealthy behaviours are often associated with pleasure in the short term but with harm in the long term (for example, lifestyle-related health conditions, unwanted pregnancy). Conversely, healthy behaviours often have long-term benefits but undesired costs in the short term (for example, effort, fatigue, stress). TST proposes that behavioural intentions are influenced by consideration of the time frame in which the behaviour will occur. Specifically this is through:

Connectedness beliefs – beliefs about the connectedness of present behaviour to later outcomes.

Temporal valuations – the values attached to outcomes occurring at different times.

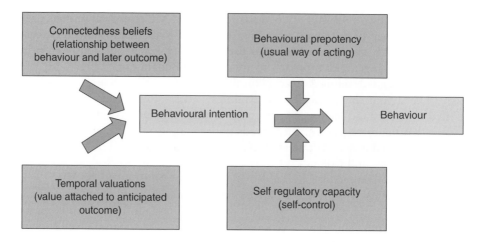

Figure 4.2   Temporal Self-regulation Theory applied to healthy choices

Hall and Fong (2007) reprinted by permission of Taylor and Francis Ltd

Example: At bedtime I may think 'Tomorrow I will go for a swim before work' – I'm thinking of the long-term benefits and all I have to do is set my alarm for 6a.m. instead of 7a.m. Tomorrow comes, and I roll over and turn off my alarm – the short-term benefits of having another hour in bed are suddenly much more attractive than the long-term benefits I had hoped to get from swimming!

The intention-behaviour gap is proposed to be influenced by an individual's:

Self-regulatory capacity – their self-control in the presence of distraction.

Behavioural prepotency – their dominant behavioural response; the response which usually takes precedence over other responses.

Behavioural prepotent responses tend to occur without conscious awareness; constant repetition over time means that they have become automatic, which explains why past behaviour is the best predictor of future behaviour (Booker and Mullan, 2013). TST is illustrated in Figure 4.2.

The theory is quite new, so research evidence is fairly limited. The predictive value of TST for maintaining a healthy lifestyle has been tested in a study of 150 undergraduates however (Booker and Mullan, 2013). Whether the participants felt 'supported by their environment' or not was assessed by asking them 'Are there any physical triggers in the environment which (positively or negatively) influence you maintaining a "healthy lifestyle"?'. Participants categorised as feeling supported by their environment were more likely to maintain a healthy lifestyle than those who felt distracted by it. In the former group, behavioural prepotency was a significant predictor of behaviour; in the latter group, behavioural prepotency, planning and response inhibition (measures of self-regulatory capacity) were predictors. The factors predicting behaviour, therefore, varied depending on the perceived supportiveness of the environment as predicted by the TST.

TST is a comprehensive theory of behaviour change since it includes consideration of rational processes (intentions), irrational processes (behaviour prepotency), internal qualities (self-regulatory capacity) and the importance of temporal context. More research is needed to develop and test behaviour change interventions utilising TST. However, a behaviour change technique which also acknowledges the role of temporal context is the use of rewards or incentives; these are discussed below.

INCENTIVES FOR BEHAVIOUR CHANGE

As has been stated, healthy choices are associated with benefits which are not usually realised until the longer term. This, coupled with the fact that a person may not believe that the benefits are certain, reduces motivation to withstand short-term costs. Provision of incentives to make healthy choices overcomes this problem by providing (near) immediate and certain reward (Giles et al., 2014). An alternative to providing an incentive is to have the individual make a 'commitment contract', whereby they deposit their own money and only receive it back once goals have been achieved. Their own money then becomes an incentive. Furthermore, a risk of loss is created in the short term which 'balances' the short-term cost of making the health behaviour change; this is considered to be effective as it is thought that people are more motivated to avoid losses than they are to achieve similarly sized gains (Halpern et al., 2012).

Most of the literature (Sutherland et al., 2008) is concerned with the provision of financial incentives. Such intervention is known as a **'health promoting financial incentive' (HPFI)** intervention. Well-conducted systematic reviews have found HPFIs to be more effective than usual care or no intervention for encouraging a range of healthy behaviour changes (n=16 studies), including smoking cessation, attendance for vaccination or screening and increasing physical activity (Giles et al., 2014) and abstinence from substance abuse (n=30 studies) (Lussier et al., 2006). The evidence also suggested that the size of the effect decreased as follow-up periods and incentive values increased, but more research is needed to test this.

Also unclear is the relative impact in the long and short term of HPFIs compared with interventions which increase intrinsic motivation to change (Sutherland et al., 2008); most health psychology theories would predict that the latter would be more effective for long-term change. Incentives may increase intrinsic motivation however – through associating a behaviour with a reward, the perceived value of the behaviour, and hence the likelihood of an individual carrying it out, may be enhanced.

In the UK, financial incentives are used across the NHS to encourage behaviour change in health professionals. Schemes such as the Quality and Outcomes Framework (QOF; BMA, 2003) and the Commissioning for Quality and Innovation scheme (CQUIN; NHS, 2006) reward GPs and Healthcare Trusts for clinical activity and health improvements made in line with government-selected indicators. For instance, under QOF, GPs have been offered incentives to offer regular annual physical health reviews to people living with a diagnosis of mental illness to help combat their increased risk of poor physical health. This is an example of an intervention being used to change the behaviour of an entire population (i.e. healthcare professionals); the following section looks briefly at population-level behaviour change interventions.

BEHAVIOUR CHANGE INTERVENTIONS – POPULATION LEVEL

Population-level interventions are 'national policies or campaigns that address the underlying social, economic and environmental conditions of a population to improve everyone's health' (NICE, 2014a). These may include mass media interventions such as leaflet, television, radio or online campaigns designed to motivate people to make healthy choices. For instance, a systematic review (Bala et al., 2013) of 11 mass media campaigns targeting smoking cessation in adults found them to be effective for changing smoking behaviour; however, study differences in methodology and quality made effects difficult to quantify.

Interventions may also be aimed at subsections of a population and are known as community-level interventions. They may be aimed at those in a particular location, those with shared interests or groups at high risk. Knowledge of the needs and preferences of the community potentially facilitates better-targeted and more effective campaigns. NICE has published guidelines for designing such interventions (NICE, 2007a).

Population-level behaviour change interventions acknowledge that we are 'social animals' – that our behaviour is influenced by the people with whom we come into contact. Interventions known as '**nudges**' utilise this fact.

Nudges (Thaler and Sunstein, 2008)

Nudges, also known as 'choice architecture interventions', involve using knowledge of human behaviour to 'nudge' people in a desired direction; in healthcare this would be towards making healthy choices. Governments or institutions, such as NHS trusts, alter environments or present choices in ways so that the healthy choice is more likely to become the default or preferred choice (Quigley, 2013). For instance, healthy eating can be encouraged by making healthy food accessible and putting unhealthy food out of reach. Internet company Google famously reduced their 2000 employees' intake of calories from M&Ms (sweets which the company provides freely to employees) by 3.1 million over the course of seven weeks simply by placing the M&Ms in opaque jars and putting dried fruit and nuts in clear jars.

Nudges may also involve creating new **social norms** by emphasising that the healthy choice is accepted or usual behaviour. For instance, a successful smoking cessation campaign aimed at Canadian young people – '15 and Falling' – emphasised that only 15 per cent of young people smoked, the nudge being that it is not 'normal' to smoke.

The use of nudges is controversial, however, with some arguing that it is inappropriate for governments and other organisations to covertly influence our choices. A lack of empirical evidence for which types of nudges in which situations are mostly likely to work has also been highlighted (Quigley, 2013).

CHAPTER SUMMARY

Methodological issues in behaviour change research were discussed. Behaviour change interventions may not be well defined in research, may lack a fully theoretical basis and may not be delivered as they were meant to be. Reporting guidelines and behaviour change systems and taxonomies have been developed to improve this.

Understanding behaviour change requires consideration of rational processes (e.g. intentions), irrational processes (e.g. behaviour prepotency, habits), internal qualities (e.g. self-regulatory capacity, self-control, motivation) and the importance of context (e.g. healthcare environment, time, rewards). A range of theories of health behaviour change was appraised.

Monitoring behaviour, receiving feedback, setting goals and action/coping planning are likely to facilitate behaviour change around making healthy choices. Behaviour change techniques that nurses, midwives and health visitors can use to help their patients were detailed.

Research evidence suggests that healthcare professionals should use every opportunity to encourage healthy choices, offer behavioural support even when they are not sure the person is interested, and review the person's progress regularly to prevent relapse.

The chapter focused on behaviour change in individuals, but population-level behaviour change was discussed briefly to highlight that individuals are influenced by those around them.

CONSOLIDATE YOUR LEARNING

 Activity: Quiz

(Answers can be found at the end of this book.)

1. Which two groups of approaches are likely to be effective to change behaviours relating to alcohol, diet, physical activity and smoking?
2. When setting goals for behaviour change, what acronym can you use to help ensure that they will be completed?
3. To what does the acronym 'OARS' refer in the context of motivational interviewing?
4. List some interventions which nurses, midwives and health visitors can use to help their patients with action planning and coping planning.

Activity: Reflection

Using behaviour change techniques to promote healthy choices

- Think about the kinds of healthy or otherwise beneficial choices you would typically like your patients or their carers to make
- Do you engage in health promotion at every opportunity? If not, why not? What gets in the way? Can you change this?
- How do you currently encourage people to make healthy choices? Do you do more than give advice? What else, if anything, do you do? How could you use the techniques in this chapter to be more effective?

FURTHER READING

Behaviour change guidance and MECC: NICE guidance (NICE, 2014) makes recommendations on individual-level behaviour change interventions for people aged 16 and over: www.nice.org.uk/guidance/ph49

An Implementation Guide and Toolkit for MECC: Using Every Opportunity to Achieve Health and Wellbeing, published by NHS Derbyshire County: www.england.nhs.uk/wp-content/uploads/2014/06/mecc-guid-booklet.pdf

The Health Trainer Handbook details evidence-based behaviour change techniques which can be used to help patients improve their health: Michie, S., Rumsey, N., Fussell, A., Hardeman, W., Johnston, M., Newman, S. and Yardley, L. (2008) *Improving Health: Changing Behaviour. NHS Health Trainer Handbook*. Manual: DH Publications.

Motivational interviewing – information on how to put MI into practice: Rollnick, S., Miller, W.R. and Butler, C.C. (2008) *Motivational Interviewing in Healthcare: Helping Patients Change Behaviour*. New York: The Guildford Press.

Nudging is discussed in detail in a popular and very readable behavioural science book: Thaler, R.H. and Sunstein, C.R. (2008) *Nudge: Improving Decisions About Health, Wealth, and Happiness*. New Haven, CT: Yale University Press.

USEFUL WEBSITE

Support Behaviour Change. RCN online learning. www.rcn.org.uk/development/practice/cpd_online_learning/support_behaviour_change

5 MANAGING ENDURING PHYSICAL SYMPTOMS

Key Learning Objectives

At the end of this chapter you will be able to explain:

- Psychological understandings of and approaches to the management of the commonly occurring and chronic symptoms of:

  o Chronic pain
  o Chest pain and palpitations
  o Breathlessness
  o Fatigue and sleep disturbance

INTRODUCTION

The focus of this chapter will be on the application of **health psychology** to the understanding and management of common and enduring physical symptoms. Symptoms such as **chronic (non-malignant) pain**, palpitations, breathlessness, fatigue and sleep disturbance are associated with a wide range of conditions or may have no medical explanation. They may be **acute** or chronic. We are concerned here with the latter, where the patient has had, or is receiving appropriate medical and nursing treatment, or no further treatment is available, but symptoms endure. The symptoms have been selected as they are very common and as nurses, midwives and health visitors, we will all encounter many people whose lives could be improved if these symptoms were better managed. Health psychology has researched and developed effective treatments for all these symptoms. Here, we will consider briefly the origins and impact of these common symptoms, but will focus on psychological explanations for them. You will be able to use the information in this chapter to help you consider the psychological perspective when caring for patients with these symptoms.

THE IMPACT OF ENDURING PHYSICAL SYMPTOMS

It is important for us as healthcare professionals to properly assess and manage common enduring symptoms as this will improve patients' quality of life and functioning. It will also lead to health economic benefits because patients with such symptoms incur high healthcare costs (Kroenke, 2003) and are often frequent users of primary care (Simon and Ormel, 1995) and emergency departments (Huffman and Pollack, 2003).

It is worth remembering that co-morbid depression and anxiety can exacerbate the perceived severity of physical symptoms (IAPT, 2008) and increase health service usage. This was discussed in detail in Chapter 2. Referral for psychological therapy of people with long-term conditions has been found to reduce emergency department attendance in these patients (De Lusignan et al., 2013). However, access to effective psychological treatment for depression and anxiety (such as cognitive behavioural therapy delivered by the government's Improving Access to Psychological Therapy – IAPT – services) is limited, waiting lists can be long and patients with physical health problems may be unwilling or unable to attend psychological therapy (IAPT, 2008; Barley et al., 2012b). Therefore, the knowledge and skills learned from Chapter 2 in managing troublesome emotions will also be useful for nurses, midwives and health visitors when helping patients to cope with their physical symptoms.

PSYCHOLOGICAL UNDERSTANDING OF ENDURING PHYSICAL SYMPTOMS

The dominant health psychology approach for understanding and managing enduring physical symptoms is the cognitive behavioural **model**, which has been discussed in relation to other aspects of health in earlier chapters. Next we discuss its application to the understanding and management of physical symptoms in general and later in relation to specific symptoms. Then an overview of other psychological approaches and techniques for managing symptoms is provided.

The Cognitive Behavioural Model Applied to Enduring Physical Symptoms

The importance of cognitive and behavioural factors in the development and maintenance of common **somatic** symptoms has been well recognised. We will discuss these in detail in relation to chronic pain, chest pain and palpitations, breathlessness, fatigue and sleep disturbance in the symptom-specific sections below. Management informed by CBT has been found to be effective for all these symptoms (Kroenke, 2003). Earlier chapters describe aspects of cognitive behavioural interventions; these are summarised in Box 5.1.

> ## Box 5.1: Cognitive behavioural interventions: typical protocol
>
> 1. Biopsychosocial assessment to identify the cause and consequences (including behavioural, emotional, cognitive, social and physiological) of the symptoms (see Chapter 1, Biopsychosocial model and Chapter 2, Thoughts, feelings, behaviour and physiology cycle). This should include assessment to ensure that the patient is receiving adequate physiological treatment.
> 2. Explanation of the cognitive model, making sure that the individual understands that their symptoms are being taken seriously.
> 3. Elicit views and beliefs and identify '**thinking errors**' (see Chapter 2) about the symptoms; for instance, using a general **illness perceptions** questionnaire (e.g. Broadbent et al., 2006, see Chapter 3 'illness perceptions') or a disease-specific questionnaire such as The York Angina Questionnaire (Furze et al., 2003).
> 4. Identify avoidance and **safety behaviours** (see Chapter 2); for instance, using daily diaries (see Chapter 7).
> 5. Challenge beliefs by highlighting past experience which does not fit with the beliefs, offering alternative evidence-based explanations, asking questions to help the person come up with their own solutions and through '**behavioural experiments**' (see Box 5.2: Behavioural experiments and Box 5.3: **Socratic questioning**).
> 6. Agree goals and action/coping plan (see Chapter 3).
> 7. Stress management advice (see Chapters 2 and 6) and relaxation training.

Although the cognitive behavioural approach to management is similar for each, particular thoughts and behaviours have been found to be associated with different symptoms. We will consider these in the following sections.

CHRONIC PAIN

Chronic pain is defined as pain without apparent biological value that has persisted beyond the normal tissue healing time, which is usually taken to be between three and six months for non-malignant pain (Mersky and Bogduk, 1994). Chronic pain is extremely common. In a large telephone survey (n=46,394), 19 per cent (ranging from 12 per cent to 30 per cent between countries) of adult respondents in 15 European countries and Israel were found to have chronic pain of moderate to severe intensity (Breivik et al., 2006); more than a quarter of adult Americans report chronic pain (National Centers for Health Statistics, 2006). Musculoskeletal pain, back pain and headache or migraine are the most common (Kroenke, 2003; National Centers for Health Statistics, 2006). Musculoskeletal pain encompasses regional, that is joints, limbs, back, neck, and more generalised pain, for instance **fibromyalgia**. Chronic gastrointestinal pain is also common (Sandler et al., 2000), including pain associated with **endometriosis** (Guo and Wang, 2006). Chronic chest pain is also common, but will be discussed separately since its association with the heart means there are special considerations.

Chronic musculoskeletal conditions account for 11 per cent of **disability-adjusted life years** (DALYs) and their impact is increasing (Murray et al., 2012). Chronic musculoskeletal pain incurs high levels of health service utilisation and costs (Kroenke, 2003; Breivik et al., 2006). Chronic pain is associated with impaired quality of life, high levels of psychological distress and reduced levels of employment (Breivik et al., 2006), which results in economic disadvantage for affected individuals and their families. The impact of chronic pain is described in the case example 'Living with chronic pain'.

 ## Case Example: Living with chronic pain

John is 48 years old. He is a qualified garage mechanic, but a few years into his career he developed lower back pain, which increased over time. John has had numerous investigations, though no definitive cause for his pain has been identified. Over the years, John has had numerous referrals for physiotherapy; unfortunately, his back pain continued to worsen. Eventually, due to his inability to perform his job, John was forced to resign. He has been unemployed for three years. He is supported by state benefits and by his wife, Ann who works part time as a supermarket checkout operator.

John and Ann live in social housing with their five children who range from age five to 17 years old. The family love animals and keep two dogs, a cat and a lizard. John takes regular analgesia which he reports 'takes the edge off' for a while. Since giving up work, John has become increasingly immobile as he has noticed that more and more types of activity cause his back pain to worsen. John's days are largely spent lying on the sofa watching television; he snacks frequently and likes a few beers to 'cheer myself up'.

As a consequence of his inactive lifestyle and poor diet, John has gained several stone over the last few years and is now overweight. This makes it even harder for him to move about and makes him feel even worse about himself. John feels bad that he barely contributes to household chores or to the care of his children and pets, but is convinced that he is unable to do more. He and his wife have frequent arguments about this. John feels that Ann is unreasonably demanding. Ann is feeling tired, stressed and increasingly tearful. She has taken a lot of time off work lately because of this and is concerned about losing her job and the implications of that for her family.

In the European survey (Breivik et al., 2006), a third of the people with chronic pain were not receiving pain management and only two per cent were receiving treatment from a pain specialist. In the UK, specialist pain clinics exist but are not widespread and vary in the support provided. A National Audit of UK Pain Services (2010–2012) has found that only half the services in England and Wales employed psychologists. Some IAPT services in England are starting to see people with chronic pain, though this is not available in all areas and the service has not yet been evaluated.

Models of Pain

For many years a medical or dualistic model of pain was accepted. This proposed a direct causal relationship between harm and hurt – tissue damage resulted in the experience of pain; the more damage, the more pain. However, this model does not explain how pain can exist in the absence of pathology or variations in the experience of pain between individuals with the same pathology.

The Gate Control Theory of Pain (GCT) (Melzack and Wall, 1982) was proposed to address these limitations. What follows is a very simplified description of this theory, for more detail please see the suggestions under Further Reading. GCT suggests that pain is experienced when pain impulses reach the brain. To reach the brain, pain impulses must pass through (hypothetical) 'gates' in the dorsal horn of the spinal cord. The central idea is that these gates can be opened or closed by both ascending physiological inputs (pain impulses) and descending psychological inputs. Psychological inputs include sensory, emotional, cognitive, experiential and genetic factors.

In chronic pain, gates may remain open once healing has occurred due to these inputs so that the individual experiences pain, even when healing has occurred. No one fully understands how this process works, nor how to control it. However, GCT (Melzack and Wall, 1982) is the only theory that accounts for both physiological and psychological aspects of the pain experience.

GCT is therefore a biopsychosocial model of pain. Although not fully explanatory, the biopsychosical model of pain now appears to be the accepted model. There is no doubt that the experience of pain is not simply a neurophysiological phenomenon, but that it also involves social and psychological factors. We will discuss psychological factors below, but the role of social factors is evidenced by observations of cultural differences in the experience of pain (Pillay et al., 2014) and the impact of the physical environment on the ability to manage pain. These factors affect an individual's emotions, behaviours and **cognition** (and vice versa) which all contribute to the pain experience.

Cognitive and Behavioural Factors in Chronic Pain

Within the biopsychosocial model of chronic pain, psychological models recognise the importance of an individual's beliefs about their pain and their ability to cope with it. In Chapter 2, we discussed 'thinking errors' or 'cognitive distortions' which may impact on emotions and functioning. Quartana and colleagues (2009) identify three common thinking errors in chronic pain:

'magnification' – Exaggerating the importance of a negative event, e.g. 'This pain is a sign that something is seriously wrong with me'.

'rumination' – Obsessive and uncontrollable preoccupation, e.g. 'I can't get this pain out of my mind'.

'helplessness' – Perceived lack of control, e.g. 'There's nothing to be done, I will always feel this way'.

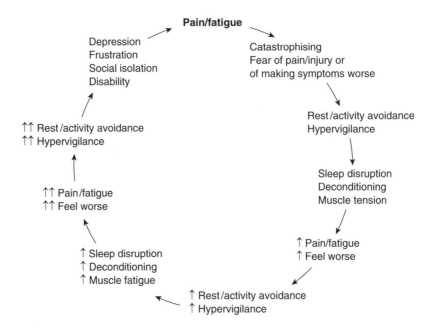

Figure 5.1   Fear-avoidance Model for pain and fatigue

Adapted from: Vlaeyen and Linton (2000)

Together these have been described as 'pain catastrophising' – an overall 'tendency to magnify or exaggerate the threat value or seriousness of pain sensations' (Quartana et al., 2009: 2).

In essence, people may believe that pain is a sign that the body is damaged and that disability is therefore inevitable (Crombez et al., 2012). Such beliefs lead to an excessive fear of pain and behavioural avoidance of activity, which the individual anticipates may cause pain. This is known as the 'Fear-avoidance Model' (Vlaeyen and Linton, 2000). People who fear pain have been found to be 'hypervigilant', that is they constantly scan their bodies for signs of pain (Crombez et al., 2012). This is associated with muscle tension, which leads to more pain. Avoidance of activity due to fear of causing pain may lead to physical deconditioning, which is in turn associated with lower tolerance of pain (Verbunt et al., 2010). Avoidance activity also means that people miss out on pleasurable experiences and social contact leading to depressed mood. Hence, pain catastrophising, measured using the pain catastrophising scale (Sullivan et al., 1995), has been found to be associated with impaired physical and psychological health and function, worse response to treatment and increased pain intensity (Sullivan et al., 2004). The Fear-avoidance cycle has also been applied to fatigue, which we will discuss below. Figure 5.1 depicts the Fear-avoidance model as applied to both pain and fatigue (Vlaeyen and Linton, 2000).

Cognitive Behavioural Management of Chronic Pain

As with all long-term conditions, self-management is key to managing chronic pain. As well as coping with pain itself, self-management involves losing weight and increasing activity to prevent or reduce disability, taking medications and adhering to treatment regimens such as physiotherapy and coping with distress. The behaviour change techniques described in Chapters 2–4 will therefore be relevant when managing patients who are experiencing chronic pain.

Specialist management of pain may involve a multidisciplinary pain management programme (PMP). The content of PMPs varies between settings and studies, but will include at least some of: psychotherapy, physiotherapy, relaxation techniques, medical treatment, patient education or vocational therapy (Scascighini et al., 2008) (see case example 'Multidisciplinary management of chronic pain').

Case Example: Multidisciplinary management of chronic pain

Let us return to the case of John detailed earlier. A new practice nurse has started at John's GP surgery. She quickly became aware, during a routine medication review, that John was experiencing multiple difficulties, was in danger of becoming seriously depressed and was concerned that John's lifestyle put him at risk of heart disease and type 2 diabetes. The practice's current treatment approach of supplying analgesia and making repeated physiotherapy referrals was clearly not working, so she organised a referral to a pain clinic.

At the pain clinic, the clinical nurse specialist carried out a full biopsychosocial assessment. This led to changes in John's medication and to further physiotherapy. This time, the physiotherapy referral was combined with a referral to a psychologist who worked with John to overcome his fears about the consequences of pain which were leading to him becoming increasingly inactive. The psychologist also helped John to consider his **motivation** to get better which gave him a reason to adhere better to his physiotherapy exercises.

The nurse taught John how to take his medication effectively and explained that he should plan activity for times when he knew that his painkillers would be having maximum effect. The multidisciplinary team agreed that John was suffering from mild depression; the treatment plan should lead to improved mood and this would be monitored. The nurse was also concerned about what John had told her about Ann's mood and encouraged him to get her to visit her GP for assessment.

The most common and effective psychological approach used within PMPs, but which can also be used as a stand-alone treatment, is cognitive behavioural therapy (CBT) (Glombiewski et al., 2010). CBT for chronic pain 'emphasises the development of personal control and self-management by means of active, structured techniques. Treatment focuses both on modifying negative thinking…and on prompting increased activity and productive functioning' (Kerns et al., 1997). Thinking errors are addressed with the aim of replacing them with more helpful beliefs, which will disrupt the fear-avoidance-disability cycle. To do this, CBT therapists may encourage the patient to identify similar situations that they have experienced in the past and ask them to see whether their current negative predictions were fulfilled then. If the patient cannot recall such a situation they may devise a 'behavioural experiment' to test the patient's assumptions (see Box 5.2: Behavioural experiments). They may also employ 'Socratic questioning' to help the patient come up with an alternative view (see Box 5.3: Socratic questioning).

Box 5.2: Behavioural experiments

A behavioural experiment is an activity that someone can do to test whether their beliefs or behaviours are helpful or unhelpful.

For instance, a common belief is 'If I become too breathless, I will faint'. This kind of belief is unhelpful as it leads to avoidance of activity which is bad for health and makes breathlessness worse.

A behavioural experiment to challenge this thinking error may involve planning to carry out an activity that would cause them to become breathless (for example, walking to the end of the road).

Planning involves deciding when, where and how to do it (e.g. they could take a friend so that they feel safe).

Before carrying out the experiment the person is asked to predict how likely they believe it is that the negative event will happen: 'It is 98 per cent likely that I will faint'.

During the event they observe exactly what happened: 'I managed to get to the end of the road. I had to use my inhaler. I felt a bit dizzy, but I did not faint'.

After the event they reflect on what the results of their experiment means in relation to their initial belief and rate how strongly they now agree with it: 'On that occasion, I was able to get breathless without fainting. It is 70 per cent likely that I will faint if I get breathless in future'.

The person may carry out a series of experiments; they will be encouraged to keep a record and share this with their CBT therapist at the next session.

Box 5.3: Socratic questioning

Socratic questioning is named after the classical Greek philosopher Socrates (470–399BC) and is a method of asking questions to stimulate discussion in order to improve understanding and to generate new ideas. In CBT it is also known as **guided discovery**. It involves the therapist asking the client a series of questions designed to help them to understand fully their current perception of a situation and to identify and consider different ways of looking at it.

A therapist may ask:

'How are you feeling?'

'What thoughts go through your head when that happens?'

'What would be bad/or good about x happening?'

'What would someone you care about say about it?'

'What could you do differently?'

'How would you advise someone in a similar situation?'

The aim is for the client to be able to apply the new information that has been brought into view to revaluate their thinking or to come up with new, more helpful ideas (Padesky, 1993).

CHEST PAIN AND PALPITATIONS

The psychological approach to managing chest pain and palpitations is similar for both, but before discussing this, let us first consider what is known about the impact and origins of each.

Chest Pain

Chest pain in coronary heart disease (CHD) may be due to angina pectoris. Angina symptoms may vary between individuals, but include painful tightness or heaviness in the chest, which may also be felt in the arms, neck, face, back or stomach. It occurs when insufficient oxygenated blood can reach the heart muscle due to coronary arteries being blocked by atheroma (fatty deposits). Angina may be predictable, in that it may be brought on by exercise or emotion (known as stable angina, typical angina or effort angina). It is commonly enduring and it is the management of enduring chest pain that is the focus here. Nevertheless, it is important to understand that angina which occurs at rest, worsens (crescendo angina) and is severe and of new onset may be an indicator of an impending heart attack. This kind of angina is termed unstable or atypical angina. Nurses should educate patients about this so that they will seek early help.

Many patients with CHD, however, also experience chest pain when no further physical treatment is available and when no current cardiological cause can be found. In a large cohort study (n=803) of primary care patients living with CHD, 44 per cent reported current chest pain despite receiving treatment for their CHD (Walters et al., 2014). Chest pain is also experienced by people with normal coronary arteries; this is known as 'non-cardiac chest pain (NCCP)' or 'non-specific chest pain'. Up to 75 per cent of people attending rapid access chest clinics may have NCCP (Sekhri et al., 2007; Debney and Fox, 2011). NCCP is associated with high levels of psychological distress, work absenteeism and impaired quality of life (Robertson et al., 2008; Parkash et al., 2009; Fass and Achem, 2011). Chest pain frequency, duration, severity, associated distress and healthcare usage is similar in people with NCCP and people with chest pain of cardiac origin (Marks et al., 2014). The impact of enduring chest pain is illustrated in the case example.

Case Example: Living with enduring chest pain

Three years ago, when he was 57 years old, Ron had a minor heart attack. He recovered well but over the last year has developed angina. His chest pain occurs during exercise and is relieved by GTN spray which his GP has prescribed. A recent **angiogram** has shown that no further intervention is necessary.

Ron is very busy in his job as a facilities manager at his local hospital. This involves moving round the hospital and visiting other sites belonging to the Trust. It is at times when he is particularly busy that Ron experiences chest pain. During an episode of chest pain, Ron becomes quite panicky and fearful. He experiences lots of worrying thoughts such as 'There is something wrong with my heart', 'I am going to have another heart attack', 'I won't be able to do my job' and even 'I might die'.

Ron has started limiting his visits to the other sites, but is worried that his manager will notice and think he isn't doing his job properly. He has started taking his GTN spray whenever he leaves the office in anticipation of developing chest pain. This overuse of his medication is causing him to feel dizzy and sick.

Ron is increasingly taking time off work because of this and is in danger of having to resign, which would have profound negative economic consequences for him and his family.

As with chest pain, people who experience palpitations may or may not have cardiac disease; we will consider this next.

Palpitations

Palpitations are experienced as rapid thumping or fluttering sensations in the chest or throat; they may last for a few seconds or for several minutes. Data are limited but one study estimated that each year around 18 per 1,000 patients visit their general practitioner (GP) with complaints of palpitations (Zweitering et al., 1996). In most of these patients, the cause will be benign (Mayou et al., 1999); for example, an adrenaline surge following emotional excitement or physical exertion, lifestyle factors (eating rich or spicy foods, excess caffeine or alcohol, recreational drugs or tobacco) or panic attacks. Palpitations are also commonly associated with anaemia, low blood pressure, thyroid problems, low blood sugar levels, dehydration, menopause, periods and pregnancy. Some medications may cause palpitations such as ventolin or thyroxine.

More seriously, palpitations may be associated with heart arrhythmias. The most common heart arrhythmia is atrial fibrillation (AF), which is a risk factor for stroke (Lane et al., 2013). Other symptoms of AF include: dizziness, breathlessness, exercise intolerance and fatigue. AF is associated with impaired quality of life (Thrall et al., 2006). However, whether or not they have a cardiac origin, palpitations are associated with increased anxiety and reduced quality of life (Hoefman et al., 2007). In some patients, impairments in quality of life endure even following treatment (Thrall et al., 2006).

Cognitive and Behavioural Factors in Chest Pain and Palpitations

Common misconceptions about heart attacks (Maeland and Havik, 1988), angina (Furze et al., 2003), and non-cardiac chest pain and palpitations (Jonsbu et al., 2010) have been identified and found to be related to worse perceived global health and recovery. Misconceptions may be around causation, disease progress or coping. For instance, an individual may believe that chest pain is due to a faulty or worn out heart, that angina causes permanent damage and that all activity that brings it on should be avoided (Furze et al., 2003).

In particular, a fear of bodily sensations has been found in both chest pain and palpitations (Jonsbu et al., 2010; Mayou et al., 1994). This leads, as in chronic pain in general, to catastrophising, i.e. assuming that chest pain or palpitations are always serious. In CHD, non-cardiac chest pain and palpitations, catastrophising and fear of bodily sensations have been found to be associated with panic and inappropriate responses such as avoidance of activity which leads to worse health and unnecessary health service use (Furze et al., 2003; Jonsbu et al., 2010) (see Figure 5.1: Fear-avoidance Model (Vlaeyen and Linton, 2000).

Cognitive Behavioural Management of Chest Pain and Palpitations

A systematic review (15 studies, n=803) found that psychological therapy, especially CBT, is of modest to moderate benefit in patients with non-cardiac chest pain (Kisely et al., 2012). There is also evidence from an RCT (n=142) of a CBT-based Angina Plan, versus a routine, practice nurse-led secondary prevention educational session, that CBT is effective for chest pain in people with diagnosed CHD (Lewin et al., 2002). An audit of the same intervention indicated reduced hospitalisations and **myocardial infarctions** pre- and post-intervention in people with refractory angina (n=271) – chronic stable angina where **revascularisation** is no longer considered feasible (Moore et al., 2007).

To date, there is only one small (n=40) RCT of CBT for palpitations (Jonsbu et al., 2011). Patients with non-cardiac chest pain and/or benign palpitations were randomised to either a three-session CBT intervention or usual GP care. The CBT intervention included '**exposure**' to physical activity to address fear of bodily sensations: patients used a treadmill and every other minute were asked to rate their perceived exertion, discomfort and worry and to describe distressing thoughts; heart rate and pulse were monitored. This gave them the opportunity to experience physical activity and to notice that it was not bad for their hearts. Patients in the intervention compared with the control group were found to report less fear of bodily sensations, avoidance of physical activity, depression and improved quality of life at the end of treatment, and at three- and 12-month follow-up.

Many of the principles of managing chest pain and palpitations are also relevant for managing breathlessness, which we consider next.

⚙️ Activity: Reflection

Think back to the case example 'Living with enduring chest pain'. You will have noted that Ron is 'catastrophising' (see Chapter 2: thinking errors): 'There is something wrong with my heart', 'I am going to have another heart attack', 'I won't be able to do my job', 'I might die'. He is also displaying **avoidance behaviours**, i.e. limiting his visits to the other sites, and safety behaviours, i.e. taking his GTN spray every time he leaves the office. All of this is having negative consequences for him in the short term, e.g. increased stress and anxiety, more chest pain, reduced activity, and in the long term, e.g. worse health, potential job loss (see Figure 2.1, p. 27 to remind yourself how these factors are interlinked).

Refer to Box 5.2. Design a behavioural experiment around Ron's safety or avoidance behaviours that Ron could do to help challenge his thinking errors.

BREATHLESSNESS

Chronic breathlessness or shortness of breath is associated with respiratory disease (for example, chronic bronchitis, emphysema, asthma), heart diseases (for example, heart failure, CHD, atrial fibrillation) and many more conditions including anaemia, panic attacks and lung cancer. Breathlessness without a detectable physiological origin occurs in 'hyperventilation syndrome' where the individual breathes too deeply or rapidly causing other symptoms including chest tightness, dizziness, tremor and paraesthesia (Jones et al., 2013).

In chronic obstructive pulmonary disease (COPD) breathlessness, along with reduced mobility and function, has been found to have the biggest impact on quality of life (Barnett, 2005; Wortz et al., 2012).

Cognitive and Behavioural Factors in Breathlessness

The impact of breathlessness is often made worse by feelings of panic. The cognitive behavioural model of panic (Clark, 1986) predicts a vicious cycle of catastrophic mis-interpretation of the cause and/or consequences of breathlessness leading to increasing fear and sympathetic arousal (see Chapter 2: physical symptoms of anxiety). Carers or others observing this response may also become fearful due to feelings of helplessness, hence inadvertently reinforcing the individual's response and escalating the process (Howard and Dupont, 2014). Behaviours resulting from this include taking too much medication (such as ventolin, which can cause tremor which, in turn, can be misinter-preted as a significant problem), constant self-monitoring for signs of breathlessness, inappropriate use of health services and avoidance of any activity which causes breath-lessness (Heslop and Foley, 2009). Reduced activity leads to deconditioning and worse health, social isolation, depression, continued smoking and a lack of motivation and energy for self-management (Livermore et al., 2010). The case example illustrates the impact of cognitive behavioural factors around breathlessness in pregnancy.

Case Example: Breathlessness in pregnancy

Danni, a 25-year-old administrator who is now 34 weeks pregnant, suffered heavy bleeding in the early stages of her pregnancy. This resulted in mild anaemia, which never resolved. Danni suffers from fatigue and breathlessness; she has been prescribed iron and folic supplements to manage her anaemia.

Danni has become increasingly anxious about the damage her anaemia may do to her baby. She regularly searches the internet for health advice and has read that her baby could be born early, underweight or may have brain damage (though this is actually only a risk in cases of severe or untreated anaemia). She has also experienced stomach disturbances from the iron tablets. She reasons that if the tablets are 'not good' for her, they can't be 'good' for her baby.

These concerns have led to her taking her supplements in an erratic way. She often feels panicky and her breathlessness seems to be increasing, she is worried about the effect of this on her baby.

Fear of becoming breathless means she has reduced her activity, she goes out less and rests more. This means she has missed out on opportunities to socialise with her friends and family.

Cognitive Behavioural Management of Breathlessness

As with all long-term symptoms and conditions, self-management is key. We have discussed self-management in Chapter 3; self-management plans for people experiencing breathlessness are likely to include intervention to stop smoking, keep active, eat healthily, maintain hydration, avoid infections, which can cause exacerbation of breathlessness especially in respiratory disease, improve breathing technique and posture, and manage emotion. Cognitive interventions for breathlessness are therefore delivered within a self-management plan adapted to the individual and taking into account the cause of breathlessness.

Cognitive intervention is aimed at challenging the misconception that all breathlessness is bad and should be avoided. Through education, behavioural experiments and opportunity to experience breathlessness in a safe environment, for instance, during pulmonary rehabilitation, the individual is taught that keeping active and confident will entail experiencing some breathlessness. The aim is that the individual will be better able to manage their breathlessness, be less restricted by it and to reduce the extent to which breathlessness is exacerbated by anxiety.

A systematic review (Coventry and Gellatly, 2008) (RCTs=3, n=165) found that CBT, when used with exercise and education, could contribute to significant reductions in anxiety and depression in patients with clinically stable and severe COPD. Also in COPD, a large (n=222), well-conducted RCT (Howard and Dupont, 2014) found that a self-help booklet with a CBT component was more effective in reducing anxiety and depression and emergency department visits than an information booklet produced by the British Lung Foundation. Both booklets were used at home over five weeks with facilitator input, which included one home visit and two telephone follow-up calls. Although the information booklet plus facilitator input was beneficial, use of the booklet with the CBT component resulted in longer-term sustained changes compared to the information only booklet.

⚙ Activity: Reflection

Think about Danni in the case example. What 'thinking errors' is she making and how might these be making her breathlessness worse? How could you help her to improve her breathlessness and stress levels? Consider how you might help challenge her unhelpful thinking through psychoeducation and behavioural experiments. Consider what else you have learnt from this book that you could use to help her improve her diet and go out more; for instance, would goal setting and action planning or motivational interviewing help (see Chapter 4)? What about some stress management or relaxation (see Chapter 6)?

People who experience breathlessness, and other enduring symptoms, commonly complain of fatigue (like Danni in the case example). We will discuss fatigue and its management in the next section.

FATIGUE

The term fatigue refers to extreme or unusual tiredness; it is sometimes considered to represent a continuum from tiredness to exhaustion (Ahlberg et al., 2003). Fatigue is very common in a range of long-term conditions, including cancer (see Useful Websites at the end of this chapter for information concerning cancer-related fatigue). It may also be an individual's primary problem as in **chronic fatigue syndrome.** The physiological mechanisms of fatigue are poorly understood (Sharpe and Wilks, 2002).

Depending on how it has been measured, the prevalence of persistent, troublesome fatigue in the general population has been reported to be from five to 20 per cent. In five to 10 per cent of primary care patients, fatigue will be the reason for their visit and it will be a secondary symptom in a further five to 10 per cent (Sharpe and Wilks, 2002).

Cognitive and Behavioural Factors in Fatigue

The Fear-avoidance Model can be applied to fatigue (White et al., 2011) as it has to pain (see Figure 5.1): fear of engaging in activity in case fatigue worsens leads to avoidance of activity which leads to deconditioning and reduced exercise tolerance. Thus inactivity is maintained, exercise intolerance increases and symptoms worsen. Catastrophising is also associated with fatigue: transient increases in symptoms may lead to catastrophic interpretations if the individual perceives fatigue to be a symptom of serious pathology.

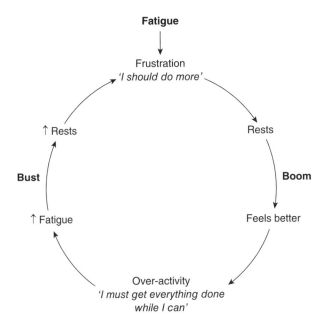

Figure 5.2   Boom and bust cycle in fatigue

Inactivity and not being able to do the things they want to may lead to feelings of frustration, especially in people who have high standards for themselves. For instance, people who have thoughts such as 'I should do more', 'I am useless because I can't do anything'. Such cognitive distortions and feelings may motivate the person to 'push themselves' or 'overdo things' during the times in which they are feeling better. Ironically, this may cause more fatigue followed by increased resting, more frustration and more 'overdoing of things'. This is known as a 'boom and bust' cycle and is depicted in Figure 5.2. 'Boom and bust' makes fatigue worse in the long run and makes it difficult for the person to develop a balanced routine (Burgess and Chalder, 2009).

Cognitive Behavioural Management of Fatigue

In patients meeting criteria for chronic fatigue syndrome (CFS), CBT and graded exercise therapy (GET) are currently recommended (NICE, 2007b). Both CBT and GET encourage people to increase their activity, though, for some years, it was uncertain whether rest or activity was the best treatment for fatigue (Price et al., 2008). In 2011, the PACE trial (n=641) (White et al., 2011) confirmed the value of exercise. It showed that, when given with specialist medical treatment, CBT and GET were more effective in improving fatigue and physical function and more cost-effective than either 'adaptive pacing therapy', where rest is balanced with activity, or specialist medical treatment alone.

In GET, individuals are helped to gradually increase physical activities, in order to reverse deconditioning from inactivity. A goal to achieve a specific level of activity will be set along with incremental, negotiated increases in duration of time spent physically active (White et al., 2011). In CBT, cognitive and behavioural factors considered to perpetuate fatigue and disability are changed through addressing unhelpful cognitions and through behavioural experiments. Typically, behavioural experiments involve establishing a routine of activity, rest and sleep, noticing what happens, then planning negotiated, incremental changes in physical and mental activity based on what they have learnt. Problem-solving techniques may be used to overcome barriers to increasing activity (White et al., 2011).

In contrast, there is limited available evidence for the effectiveness of interventions for the management of fatigue associated with a physical condition, though a systematic review in rheumatoid arthritis (Cramp et al., 2013) found some evidence for exercise and psychosocial interventions. Similarly, a systematic review (Payne et al., 2012) examining interventions to manage fatigue (and/or unintentional weight loss) in the advanced stage of progressive illnesses including advanced cancer, heart failure, lung failure, cystic fibrosis, multiple sclerosis, motor neurone disease, Parkinson's disease, dementia and AIDS found a lack of robust evidence. RCTs are clearly needed to determine the best management plan for fatigue associated with physical ill health.

Whatever approach is used and whatever the cause of the fatigue, however, a **shared decision-making** approach should be taken when setting goals and planning changes. This is especially important when helping people to manage symptoms of unknown origin. People who have not been provided with an explanation for their symptoms which they find acceptable may be especially sensitive to implications that their problems are 'all in their head'. This is also likely to be the case for people who are convinced that their symptoms result from a condition that is yet to be detected. Everyone needs to feel that their concerns are being taken seriously before they will engage in treatment. It helps if the healthcare professional considers the individual to be the expert in their own body.

SLEEP DISTURBANCE

Sleep disturbances include insomnia, which refers both to difficulties in falling and in staying asleep, and early morning waking with difficulty going back to sleep (Montgomery and Dennis, 2002). In the adult general population, it is estimated that nine to 15 per cent report chronic insomnia, with reports rising to 25 to 50 per cent in the elderly; in addition 25 to 30 per cent report transient insomnia (Benca, 2005). Sleep disturbance is related to psychological distress, fatigue and poor concentration. It results in absenteeism, premature mortality, reduced quality of life and high healthcare costs (Saddichha, 2010). Sleep disturbance is also a common problem throughout childhood; it can persist for many years and has a negative impact on both children and their families (Tikotzky and Sadeh, 2010). While sleep-disturbed adults may be slowed down and sluggish, sleep disorder children may overcompensate and speed up causing more tiredness and sleep disturbance for themselves and their carers. This is illustrated in the case example.

Case Example: Sleep disturbance in a child

Joseph is nine years old and has never been a 'good sleeper'. He has mild learning difficulties and has recently been diagnosed with **attention deficit hyperactivity disorder (ADHD)**.

His parents like to wait until he appears tired before putting him to bed. This means that his bed time can vary nightly by several hours. Joseph has an elaborate bedtime ritual involving listening to music and reading a single story several times. His parents, Celia and Gareth, generally have to return to his room several times each evening to settle him. They often give in to his demands for 'just a short story', which inevitably leads to them having to read the same story several times. Joseph insists on having his bedroom light left on all night. During the night Celia and Gareth are usually woken around 3 a.m. by the sound of Joseph jumping on his bed. He is very difficult to settle after that, and, more often than not, one parent will stay up with him until the morning.

At school, Joseph is hyperactive and inattentive in lessons. He is often aggressive towards other children. This is causing tension between the school and his parents, as well as between his parents and other parents who feel Joseph is disrupting their child's education.

Celia gave up work a few years ago as she felt too tired to work. She complains of constant tiredness. Gareth has a long commute, he would like to work locally but would probably have to take a salary cut which the family can't afford while Celia is not working. Tensions between the couple are running high; they can't understand why their child needs less sleep than other children and feel that 'life is unfair'.

Cognitive and Behavioural Factors in Sleep Disturbance

Lundh and Broman (2000) suggest that sleep disturbance may result from two processes:

1. Sleep-interpreting processes – misperceptions about sleep ('I must have eight hours sleep to stay healthy'), as well as dysfunctional beliefs, expectations and attributions concerning sleep and the causes ('My insomnia is a sign of a serious medical problem') and consequences ('If I don't get enough sleep I will give a poor presentation tomorrow and I will be kicked off my course') of poor sleep. Carers of children who experience sleep disturbance may hold similar unhelpful beliefs around their child's lack of sleep.
2. Sleep-interfering processes – cognitive, emotional and physiological arousal-producing processes that interfere with sleep such as anxiety, worry, pain or other symptoms.

The two processes may mutually reinforce each other. For example, a belief that insufficient sleep will have disastrous consequences (catastrophising) is likely to arouse anxiety, which further disrupts sleep. Anxiety may reinforce the original cognitive distortion or generate others (for example – 'I just can't sleep, there must be something wrong with me'), which create more anxiety – hence there is a vicious cycle of sleep disturbance (Broman and Lundh, 2003).

Other factors found to be implicated in disturbed sleep include conditioned bedtime arousal, irregular sleep schedules and excessive time spent in bed (Edinger et al., 2001).

Management of Sleep Disturbance

Pharmacological interventions have unpleasant side effects and evidence for their effectiveness is limited (Bootzin and Epstein, 2011). Multicomponent cognitive behavioural therapy for insomnia or sleep disturbance is now a well-established treatment (Morin et al., 2006). Treatments vary, but common components are detailed in Box 5.3.

Box 5.3: CBT for insomnia

Sleep education – for instance, providing information around sleep requirements, sleep and aging, sleep loss, and **circadian rhythms**.

Setting and planning to adhere to **sleep hygiene** rules – for instance, cutting down on caffeine, alcohol and smoking, not going to bed hungry, making sure the bedroom is non-stimulating by keeping it dark, quiet and not too hot and having a relaxing pre-sleep routine (winding down).

Sleep restriction – restricting time in bed to actual sleep time, getting up when awake to break the pattern of sleeplessness.

Stimulus control – making sure that the bed is associated with sleep and sexual activity only by not using it for other activities such as working, watching television, planning, worrying or any other activity which is not compatible with sleep. This avoids the problem of conditioning (see 'relaxation' below) where the bed becomes associated with not being able to sleep.

Cognitive restructuring – changing or replacing unhelpful thoughts around the causes and consequences of poor sleep.

Relaxation therapy – reducing arousal through relaxation (see below).

(adapted from Dalrymple et al., 2010)

Though this appears to be a time-consuming and specialist intervention, a RCT (n=101) found that CBT for insomnia delivered in five sessions in small groups by primary care nurses was more effective than treatment as usual delivered by general practitioners (Espie et al., 2005).

So far we have focused on cognitive behavioural models of and treatments for enduring physical symptoms. The role of a number of other psychological constructs has also been considered; let us look at this next.

⚙ **Activity: Reflection**

Consider Joseph from the case example. From what you have learnt about sleep disturbance, how could you approach starting to help the family? In particular, consider whether
there are any unhelpful beliefs and problems with sleep hygiene which may be contributing to Joseph, Celia and Gareth's problems. What could be done to address them?

PSYCHOLOGICAL CONSTRUCTS STUDIED IN RELATION TO ENDURING PHYSICAL SYMPTOMS

The cognitive behavioural approach to understanding and managing common
enduring symptoms is the dominant health psychology model, but other psychological constructs have also been applied, namely **self-efficacy** (see Chapter 3), locus
of control (Rotter, 1966) and conditioning. These are detailed briefly next.

Self-efficacy: In chronic pain, high self-efficacy – a strong belief within an individual that they can cope with their pain – has been found to be associated with
reporting lower pain intensity (Rahman et al., 2008). Higher levels of self-efficacy
in COPD have been found to be associated with lower reported levels of breathlessness (Simpson and Jones, 2013).

Locus of control: According to locus of control theory (Rotter, 1966) people with
an 'internal locus of control' believe that they can control what happens to them,
whereas people with an 'external locus of control' believe that external factors
such as fate, chance or others are more important. Patient-controlled analgesia
(PCA) is designed to give patients a greater sense of control over their pain, in
that they can access analgesia when they need it and can control the dose they
require rather than waiting for a clinician to have time to attend them or for a
dose scheduled for a specific time. Greater satisfaction has been reported for PCA
compared to on demand analgesia administered by others (Chang et al., 2004).
Furthermore, it has been found that patients with an external locus of control
report more pain and greater dissatisfaction with PCA then those with an internal
locus of control (Johnson et al., 1989; Thomas et al., 1995).

Conditioning: This is a learning process which explains the role of experience in
symptom perception. 'Classical conditioning' is the process whereby repeated pair-
ing of a neutral stimulus with another stimulus, which is associated with a specific
response, leads to that response becoming associated with the previously neutral
stimulus. For instance, an inappropriately conditioned fatigue sensation could be
a cause of chronic fatigue: in a small experimental study (Ishii et al., 2013), participants (n=19) heard the sound of a metronome while repeating fatigue-inducing
memory tasks. Later, just the sound of the metronome was found to induce a feeling of fatigue and an associated physiological response. Larger studies are needed
to confirm this though. In 'operant conditioning' the likelihood of a specific

behaviour is increased or decreased through positive or negative reinforcement. Eventually, the individual will associate the pleasure or displeasure of the reinforcement with the behaviour. For instance, breathlessness may be associated with behaviours such as reducing activity, gasping, staying off work. These behaviours may be positively reinforced through receipt of sympathy, attention or time off. Such reinforcement may then increase perceived breathlessness.

As well as the theory-based interventions and models discussed so far, there are other more simple strategies which may be of use in coping with enduring physical symptoms. We detail these briefly next.

SIMPLE STRATEGIES FOR COPING WITH ENDURING PHYSICAL SYMPTOMS

The following techniques are popular and widely used, but there is a lack of evidence for how and in what situation they may work. However, they may work through reducing cognitive, emotional and physiological arousal which is interfering with functioning, by reducing hypervigilance for symptoms or by increasing self-efficacy by increasing the individual's sense that they are taking an active stance and so are in control. For these reasons, nurses, midwives and health visitors may find it useful to share the techniques detailed below with patients, but should do so with caution and not in place of evidence-based interventions.

Relaxation: There are numerous techniques and effectiveness is likely to vary with the individual. Individuals can try different techniques and find which suits them. Techniques include: progressive muscle relaxation, diaphragmatic breathing, autogenic training, electromyography biofeedback, meditation, yoga, hypnosis and **mindfulness**. Mindfulness is discussed in Chapter 7; there are a range of freely available resources describing the other techniques (see Further Reading).

Imagery: Refers to mental sensory experiences (sights, sounds, feelings, smells or tastes) and can be contrasted with cognitions, which are in the form of verbal language (Berna et al., 2012). Therapeutic imagery is the deliberate conjuring of sensory experiences, rather than the spontaneous images that occur in response to specific situations, thoughts or feelings. Imagery may be induced by the person alone or through guided imagery where someone else progressively describes the image. Imagery may be used to induce relaxation, for instance, by imaging oneself to be in a calm, peaceful place. It may be used to create a sense of control, for instance, when the individual imagines white blood cells attacking a tumour or source of infection or imagines positive energy flowing in and out of their body.

Distraction: Involves deliberate shifting of attention away from the symptom and focusing instead on something else, for instance, through reading, watching television or listen to music. This is hard to sustain however and is more likely to be useful for short periods and when the alternative focus is particularly absorbing.

CHAPTER SUMMARY

Enduring physical symptoms, such as chronic pain, chest pain, palpitations, breathlessness, fatigue and disturbed sleep, may or may not have a known physiological origin. In either instance, they cause physical and psychological suffering and impact negatively on quality of life.

Cognitive behavioural approaches to treatment which address cognitive distortions around the symptom, its cause and its consequences and which promote an active coping response have been found to improve the impact of enduring physical symptoms.

Different cognitive distortions or unhelpful thoughts have been identified for different symptoms. Catastrophising and 'fear-avoidance' are common and have been well researched.

Other relevant psychological constructs and techniques were discussed and are useful to understand, but there has been less research around them compared with cognitive behavioural models.

CONSOLIDATE YOUR LEARNING

 Activity: Quiz

(Answers can be found at the end of this book.)

1. The Fear-avoidance Model (Vlaeyen and Linton, 2000) has been used to explain health behaviour associated with which common, enduring symptoms?
2. The experience of chest pain, palpitations and breathlessness are often associated with panic. Which thinking error is commonly associated with panic?
3. Which two psychological processes are proposed to interfere with sleep?
4. In relation to fatigue, what is meant by the 'boom and bust' cycle?

 Activity: Reflection

Identifying and addressing cognitive distortions to help patients manage their enduring physical symptoms

Cognitive behavioural therapy training involves intensive study and hours of practice. However, awareness of common thinking errors associated with enduring symptoms and the impact on the patient can help us as nurses, midwives and health visitors to educate and reassure them and to ensure that they receive appropriate help.

(Continued)

(Continued)

- Think of at least two patients who you know are coping with enduring physical symptoms. Try to pick one who seems to be coping well and one who seems to be coping less well
- What differences are there in the way they describe their symptoms and their lives?
- What strategies, if any, do they use?
- Could you use the information you have discovered to help the patient who is coping less well?

FURTHER READING

Detailed textbook on using CBT for distress in physical illness: Sage, N., Sowden, M., Chorlton, E. and Edeleanu, A. (2008) *CBT for Chronic Illness and Palliative Care: A Workbook and Toolkit*. London: John Wiley and Sons.

Comprehensive pain resource which covers the biology of pain, pain management across the life-course and key topics such as acute pain, cancer pain and pharmacology: Wright, S. (2014) *Pain Management in Nursing Practice*. London: Sage.

USEFUL WEBSITES

More details about the symptoms discussed in this chapter and related conditions:

Pain, The British Pain Society: www.britishpainsociety.org/

Breathlessness, The British Lung Foundation: www.blf.org.uk/

Chest pain, The British Heart Foundation: www.bhf.org.uk/

Sleep, The National Sleep Foundation: sleepfoundation.org/

Fatigue, Oncology Nursing Society (cancer-related fatigue, but similar principles apply whatever the cause of fatigue): www.ons.org/

An excellent self-help resource for breathlessness and anxiety written by clinical health psychologist Jane Hutton: www.kcl.ac.uk/ioppn/depts/pm/research/imparts/Quick-links/Self-Help-Materials/Breathlessness-and-anxiety.pdf

Relaxation, multiple resources exist: recorded guided meditation and other relaxation exercises at www.getselfhelp.co.uk, where CBT informed help can also be found for a range of problems: www.getselfhelp.co.uk/mobile/relax.htm

6 LOOKING AFTER YOURSELF

Key Learning Objectives

At the end of this chapter you will be able to explain:

- Wellbeing
- Risk factors for impaired health and wellbeing in health professionals
- Work stress and burnout
- Positive psychology
- Resilience and flourishing
- The link between wellbeing and health
- Ways to improve wellbeing
- Mindfulness

INTRODUCTION

In this chapter, we will consider work- and lifestyle-related risk factors for impaired health and wellbeing in health professionals. We will explore the concept of wellbeing in depth. We need to understand this as clinicians' health and wellbeing can not only have negative personal impact, but may also affect patients. We will then consider ways to improve wellbeing. The information in this chapter will help us as nurses, midwives and health visitors to help ourselves, but we can also use it to help our patients and their relatives to improve their wellbeing. As healthcare professionals, we need to understand how to improve wellbeing in order to be able to provide truly holistic care.

RISK FACTORS FOR IMPAIRED HEALTH AND WELLBEING IN HEALTH PROFESSIONALS

It is well known that work- and lifestyle-related factors are associated with ill health and reduced wellbeing. Nurses, midwives and health visitors face the same challenges as the rest of the population. However, there are particular aspects of the roles of health professionals that may put us particularly at risk of work-related stress or of unhealthy lifestyles. Being stressed and/or unhealthy may impact both on the clinician and on those for whom they are responsible. We will look at work stress and physical health separately, although we know from Chapter 2 that thoughts, feelings, physiology and behaviours are very much interlinked.

WORK STRESS AND HEALTH PROFESSIONALS

Psychological conceptualisations of stress were discussed in Chapter 2; for practical purposes here we will use the term 'stress' to refer to any experience of psychological distress. 'Work stress' will refer to psychological distress associated with an individual's job role. '**Burnout**' is an extreme form of work stress which has been studied in nurses and others working in caring professions; it is defined in Box 6.1: Burnout.

Research has identified a range of work-related predictors of stress and burnout across professions, these include: excessive workload, time pressure, role conflict or ambiguity, lack of support from colleagues, lack of control and **autonomy**, perceived lack of intrinsic or extrinsic reward (Maslach et al., 2001) and requirement to display or suppress emotions (Zapf et al., 2001). The last has been termed 'emotion work' or 'emotional labour' and may be especially relevant to those in caring roles, such as nursing (Zapf, 2002).

Several measures of nursing-related stress exist, and French and colleagues (2000) used factor analysis of their items, plus items identified through focus groups, to define nine nursing-related stressors: dealing with death and dying, conflict with physicians, inadequate preparation to deal with others' emotional needs, problems with peers, problems with supervisors, workload, uncertainty concerning treatment, dealing with patients and their families and feeling discriminated against (on the basis of age, gender and ethnicity). Of course, individuals will respond differently to each stressor, but it is possible that emotion work coupled with organisational problems is especially likely to lead to high levels of burnout (Zapf, 2002).

Box 6.1: Burnout

First used to describe workers' reactions to the **chronic** stress experienced in relation to job-related distressing interpersonal interactions (Freudenberger, 1974). Care-giving roles involve particularly stressful interpersonal interactions, which is why burnout is associated with nursing and related professions.

Symptoms include (Maslach et al., 2001):

- Overwhelming emotional exhaustion: feeling 'overextended' and depleted of emotional and physical resources
- Sense of inefficacy and lack of accomplishment: feelings of being incompetent or unproductive
- Cynicism and detachment for the job: sometimes known as 'depersonalisation', a negative, callous or excessively detached response, related to '**compassion fatigue**'

Figure 6.1 shows how these symptoms are interlinked with burnout becoming a vicious circle.

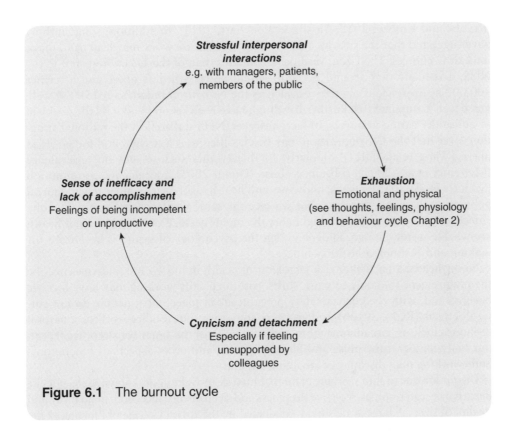

Figure 6.1 The burnout cycle

Organisation problems are often revealed through staff surveys. In the UK, the National Health Service (NHS) Staff Survey is conducted annually by the government with the aim of helping NHS organisations to 'review and improve staff experience so that staff can provide better patient care' (NHS England, 2014). In 2014, 624,000 full- and part-time staff from a range of job roles within 287 NHS organisations were invited to participate; 42 per cent responded (n=255,000). The survey found (as in previous years) that stress is common: 39.5 per cent of respondents reported experiencing work-related stress in the last 12 months.

The survey was not all bad news: 73 per cent felt supported in a personal crisis, 68 per cent reported always being enthusiastic about their jobs and 74 per cent of staff said that time passed by quickly when they were working. However, the problem of work stress for nurses, midwives and health visitors working at all levels and in a range of settings has been well documented (McVicar, 2003; Collins, 2006; Riahi, 2011; Wallbank and Hatton, 2011). Similarly, research has investigated the association between nursing and physical health; we will consider this now.

NURSING AND PHYSICAL HEALTH

Risks to nurses' musculoskeletal health from heavy lifting and static load (non-dynamic working positions such as when bathing patients) are well documented

(Knibbe and Knibbe, 2012; Yassi and Lockhart, 2013). In addition, some authors have suggested that the stresses and strains of healthcare work may lead us to make unhealthy choices. The UK government estimates that 'of the 1.2 million staff in the NHS, it is likely that around 300,000 would be classified as obese and a further 400,000 as overweight'. Initiatives, such as the *Nursing Standard*'s (2015) 'Eat well, nurse well' campaign (see Further Reading), have been set up to address the problem of unhealthy eating in nurses. In fact, however, NHS staff reflect the national situation: over half the UK population may be classified as overweight and a quarter as obese (Wang et al., 2011). Similarly, for behaviours such as smoking prevalence (McKenna et al., 2001), substance abuse (Dunn, 2005) and alcohol consumption (Schluter et al., 2011), nurses, midwives and health visitors are similar to the general population. It seems therefore that we face the same challenges in making healthy choices as everyone else. This highlights the main message of this book: that health knowledge is not enough, understanding the psychology of health is important for making and sustaining healthy choices.

Nevertheless, a particular risk factor for ill health in nurses and midwives may be the requirement for some to work shifts. Although shift working may have lifestyle benefits and, with the correct safety precautions in place, most people do not suffer ill effects (RCN, 2012b), it does carry some risk. Our bodies work to a natural 24-hour clock or '**circadian rhythm**', which regulates the times we sleep, wake, eat, our body temperature, pulse and blood pressure, and other aspects of functioning. Shift working may disrupt our circadian rhythm.

Disruption due to shift working of our habitual sleep-wake cycle, known as sleep-wake disturbance, can result in excessive sleepiness and sleep disturbance, both in quantity and quality of sleep. A large-scale survey conducted by the Royal College of Nursing in the UK suggested that nurses find shift working tiring and that very few manage to get the number or length of breaks they need (RCN, 2012c). Prolonged sleep disturbance has also been associated with cancer (Straif et al., 2007), cardiovascular disease (Puttonen et al., 2010), depression (Driesen et al., 2011) and an increased susceptibility to minor illnesses such as colds and gastroenteritis (Health and Safety Executive, 2006).

Now let us consider why understanding the impact of nursing on our physical and emotional health is important.

THE IMPORTANCE OF HEALTH AND WELLBEING IN HEALTH PROFESSIONALS

Clearly, prolonged stress and unhealthy lifestyles are as bad for nurses, midwives and health visitors as they are for anyone else, but nurses' wellbeing has been found to be lower than the general working population (RCN, 2005). Sickness absence within healthcare professions is high; costs to the UK NHS are thought to be around 1.4 billion per year (NHS Employers, 2014). Apart from ambulance staff, nurses, midwives and health visitors in the UK have the highest rate of sickness absence. In 2013–14, rates of 4.72 per cent were recorded for qualified nursing, midwifery and health visiting staff in NHS organisations, though this has been falling in recent years (HSCIC, 2014). A large review of NHS staff (Boorman, 2009) found that half of all sickness absence was accounted for by musculoskeletal disorders and over a quarter was accounted for by stress, depression and anxiety.

Poor health and wellbeing in nurses, midwives and health visitors also results in 'presenteeism'. This is where staff attend work despite being unfit to contribute. Pressures to do so may be self-directed, for instance when staff who are unfit turn up for work out of guilt brought on by awareness of the impact of their absence on patients and colleagues. Alternatively, staff may feel intimidated by managers, or anxious that poor attendance records may be used against them in future staffing decisions. Whatever the reason, presenteeism can result in poor performance and may be dangerous to the staff member's health or to patients; for instance, when staff come to work with an infectious condition.

Studies have also shown that the health and wellbeing of healthcare professionals is linked to service quality and to patient experience (Boorman, 2009; Maben et al., 2012). In the UK, the Francis Inquiry (Francis, 2013), which investigated poor patient outcomes in the Mid-Staffordshire NHS Foundation Trust, reported that when nurses feel unable to do their job properly they can withdraw and behave in negative and defensive ways which can lead to poor practice. In a large, mixed methods study using observation and patient and staff surveys and interviews, Maben and colleagues (2012) found a clear relationship between staff wellbeing and staff-reported patient care performance and patient-reported patient experience. In this work, staff wellbeing was seen as an antecedent of patient experience rather than a consequence of care performance.

The physical health of health professionals may also impact indirectly on patients. Sleep disturbance due to shift patterns and the resulting sleepiness at work can result in nursing errors and impair patient safety (Dorrian et al., 2006, 2008). Less directly, an unhealthy appearance may reduce a healthcare professional's credibility: 37 per cent of Mori poll respondents would not accept health advice from a healthcare professional who appeared to have an unhealthy lifestyle (Ipsos Mori, 2009). Similarly, clinicians may be less likely to offer behaviour change support to patients if they themselves are struggling with the behaviour (Vickers et al., 2007). For instance, a review of 20 studies found that doctors who were current smokers had a 17 per cent increased risk of not advising their patients to quit compared with never-smokers (Duaso et al., 2014).

As healthcare professionals our health and wellbeing is therefore important for us personally, for our patients and for the organisations in which we work. The case example 'The importance of health professional health and wellbeing' puts this in context.

Case Example: The importance of health and wellbeing in health professional

Anita trained as a child nurse because she loved children, liked working with people, was interested in health and wanted to 'make a difference'. After qualifying she worked on a general surgery ward. She quickly had children of her own and then spent years working nights to fit around them. Once they were teenagers she took a job on a specialist neurosurgical ward where she could work office hours.

(Continued)

(Continued)

In the years when she was juggling work and childcare, Anita found she had little time to look after herself. Her meal times were irregular and she would often eat unhealthy convenience food to save time. Anita always planned to do something about the weight that was piling on but never seemed to have the time or energy.

Though working office hours improved how tired Anita had been feeling, her increasing weight made the physical demands of her busy job harder and harder. She developed low back pain and had to take anti-inflammatories, but these made her feel sick and upset her stomach. She knew she should seek alternative treatment, but couldn't see how she could fit physiotherapy appointments into her busy life, let alone practise the exercises, so she didn't bother.

The emotional burden of her work on the neurosurgical ward was also high. She witnessed a lot of pain and death and sometimes felt that she couldn't listen to 'another sad story'. On top of this she had to deal regularly with stressed and angry parents. It was hard not to take it personally when they seemed to blame her for their child being sick.

At the end of each day Anita was tired and irritable. She would snap at her teenage children then console herself by eating chocolate and drinking wine. This added to her weight problems, her back pain worsened and her mood dropped. The ward was very busy and, Anita felt, poorly managed. Consequently (she believed) there was a high staff turn-over. Having to show agency staff what to do added to Anita's workload. With many demands to satisfy, Anita felt that the care she gave was always rushed. She found herself feeling irritable with her patients and with their parents and it took all her energy to maintain her patience. This made her feel bad about herself as she knew she wasn't being the kind of nurse she wanted to be.

Recommendations have been made as to how organisations should support staff health and wellbeing (HSE, 2007; Maben et al., 2012). However, as employees we may have limited control over how or whether recommendations are implemented. We can, however, take more control over our own health and wellbeing. Even in the context of demanding work with irregular hours, we can apply the behaviour change techniques detailed throughout this book to help us make and sustain healthy choices.

⚙️ Activity: Reflection

What healthy changes do you, or Anita in the case example, need to make to be and feel healthier? Which of the behaviour change techniques that you have learnt about could you use to help make one or more of these changes? What would you advise Anita?

There is also a considerable body of research which can help us to improve our wellbeing. Before discussing this research, let us first explore how psychologists and other researchers have defined this construct.

WELLBEING

Objective Versus Subjective Wellbeing

There are no universally agreed definitions of the terms 'objective wellbeing' and 'subjective wellbeing'. Objective wellbeing has been measured in terms of variables external to the individual which are important for human functioning and life quality; for instance, income level, material conditions or job security. Which factors are measured will depend on which are valued by whoever is making the measurement. However, it has been well established, through research conducted by both psychologists and economists and discussed in popular science books, that how people feel – their subjective wellbeing – is influenced by more than external variables such as wealth (Layard, 2005). For instance, research from the United States, Britain and Japan shows that despite average incomes having doubled in the last 50 years, people are no happier today (Layard, 2005: 3).

That there is more to wellbeing than money is good news for nurses and other healthcare professionals since our jobs are unlikely to make us rich! Instead, there may be other factors which are more under our control and on which we can work to improve our subjective wellbeing. Psychological research has sought to identify these factors, but first let us look at how subjective wellbeing has been defined. (Note: to aid reading and since subjective rather than objective wellbeing is of primary interest to psychologists, following the next subheading, the term 'wellbeing' will be used to mean 'subjective wellbeing'.)

SUBJECTIVE WELLBEING

Early psychological research (Bradburn, 1969) identified that subjective wellbeing was of primary importance for how well individuals coped with daily difficulties. However, the term 'wellbeing' was poorly defined and was treated as synonymous with 'happiness' (Dodge et al., 2012). Latterly, happiness, or more generally 'positive affect', has been considered only one aspect of wellbeing. Wellbeing may also incorporate 'life satisfaction', that is an individual's cognitive sense of satisfaction with life (Diener and Suh, 1997).

Also treated as synonymous with wellbeing, in a variety of disciplines, is the term 'quality of life' (QoL) (Dodge et al., 2012). Many definitions of QoL exist. The most well known is probably that of the World Health Organization which says that QoL is:

an individual's perception of their position in life in the context of the culture and value systems in which they live and in relation to their goals, expectations, standards and concerns. It is a broad ranging concept affected in a complex way by the person's physical health, psychological state, personal beliefs, social relationships and their relationship to salient features of their environment (World Health Organization, 1997).

However, it has also been argued that QoL is only one dimension of wellbeing (Dodge et al., 2012).

While there remains no universally agreed definition of wellbeing, three broad dimensions which encompass all of the above are increasingly accepted as constituting wellbeing. These are: life evaluation, hedonic wellbeing and eudemonic wellbeing (Steptoe et al., 2015).

Life evaluation: refers to how people perceive the overall quality or goodness of their lives. It encompasses life satisfaction and aspects of quality of life.

Hedonic wellbeing: refers to experienced feelings or moods. Both positive and negative affect are important for wellbeing. Positive emotions, such as happiness, and negative emotions, such as sadness or anger, are not wholly inversely related, that is, they can exist alongside each other. Each provides information about the individual's emotional state and each should be measured to provide a comprehensive assessment of wellbeing. The concept of hedonic wellbeing derives from a philosophic perspective which suggests that maximising one's pleasurable moments is the pathway to happiness (Henderson and Knight, 2012).

Eudemonic wellbeing: refers to an individual's judgement about the meaning and purpose of their life. It derives from Aristotle's idea of 'eudaimonia' and the related philosophical perspective that living a life of virtue and actualising one's inherent potentials is the way to wellbeing (Henderson and Knight, 2012).

The discipline of psychology has always been concerned with the study of human wellbeing, nevertheless it has been noted that the focus of psychology has been on psychology (Seligman and Csikszentmihalyi, 2000). This realisation led to the formation, by American psychologist Martin Seligman, of the **positive psychology** movement, which we will consider next.

POSITIVE PSYCHOLOGY

Positive psychology is concerned with positive human functioning; not just how people overcome adversity but what makes life worth living (Seligman and Csikszentmihalyi, 2000). Positive psychology constructs such as strengths, **values**, adaptation, positive affect and disposition, thriving and growth were studied by psychologists before the advent of positive psychology, but Seligman and Csikszentmihalyi (2000) were the first psychologists to organise the field. They did this around three themes: positive experience, positive personality, and positive communities and institutions (Aspinwall and Tedeschi, 2010). There has been exponential growth in positive psychology research since its inception, much of which is beyond the scope of this book – for the interested reader numerous texts and websites discussing positive psychology are available.

Here we will focus on two key positive psychology constructs that are relevant to the wellbeing of nurses, midwives and health visitors. These are 'resilience' and 'flourishing'.

Resilience: is essentially the ability to 'bounce back' after a setback. More formally, in the context of nursing, it has been defined as 'the ability of an individual to adjust to adversity, maintain equilibrium, retain some sense of control over their environment, and continue to move on in a positive manner' (Jackson et al., 2007: 3). A systematic review of studies concerned with resilience and workplace adversity in nursing (Jackson et al., 2007) suggests that nurses can work to strengthen their personal resilience. Strategies such as: building positive and nurturing professional relationships, maintaining positivity, developing emotional insight, achieving life balance and spirituality and becoming more reflective were found to be important. In addition, in an online discussion between 11 midwives self-reported to be resilient (Warren and Hunter, 2014) learning to pre-empt stressful situations and take action to avoid these was identified as resilience building. Past positive experience of coping with adversity was also highlighted; the benefits of such '**mastery experiences**' have been described in earlier chapters in relation to coping with LTCs for which personal resilience is also needed. The case example 'A resilient midwife' illustrates how one person copes with difficulties at work.

 ## Case Example: A resilient midwife

Julie is a newly qualified midwife on a busy labour ward. As a third-year student she had felt confident in her abilities and was looking forward to qualifying. However, rather than providing actual support, her Trust's preceptorship scheme has turned out to be a bit of a 'paper exercise' and she now finds that she has really been thrown in at the deep end. Night shifts are particularly busy and she often feels quite terrified when at work. Paperwork is also proving to be more of a burden than she anticipated and she resents that it takes her away from giving the quality of care that she wants to the women. Recent harsh treatment from her manager over uncompleted paperwork upset her a great deal.

Julie admits to being a bit of a worrier; however, she also sees herself as someone who doesn't give up easily and who can bounce back from adversity. She is quickly becoming aware of the challenges of her job. Making time to check carefully what she and others are doing helps her to feel confident that her practice is safe.

Julie also feels lucky to be part of a team where she has identified several like-minded individuals. Talking through her feelings with them is helpful for her, and she has been surprised to find that even quite experienced staff share similar anxieties. This is reassuring for her as she realises that her fears are 'natural' and can be managed. Making the effort to reflect with her colleagues on positive experiences too reminds her of the benefits of being a midwife and of the difference she can make to women and their babies.

When problems arise, Julie has learnt to try to make a plan to deal with them so that she doesn't lie awake worrying at night. Her colleagues have made her aware of the importance of 'leaving work behind' and of maintaining her outside interests so that she does not become overwhelmed with work concerns. At home, she tells her husband about her shift as a way of 'letting go', but she always makes the effort to change the conversation to focus on other things. This reminds her that there is more to life than work and that being a midwife is only one aspect of herself; that way, when things are tough at work, she can draw strength by focusing on the parts of her life that are going well.

> ### ⚙ Activity: Reflection
>
> What strategies do you currently use to build your personal resilience? Some strategies may feel natural, but are there others which Julie uses or from those listed above that you could develop?

Flourishing: According to 'the father of positive psychology', Martin Seligman, flourishing is the ultimate state of wellbeing: *'I used to think that the topic of positive psychology was happiness. I now think that the topic of positive psychology is wellbeing, that the gold standard for measuring wellbeing is flourishing, and that the goal of positive psychology is to increase flourishing'* (Seligman, 2011: 13). Flourishing is considered to occur when both hedonic and eudemonic wellbeing are present (Henderson and Knight, 2012), that is when people both feel good and have a sense of value and purpose. In his book *Flourish* (2011), Seligman details his theory of, and sets out the evidence for, which elements of wellbeing he believes are important to develop for a flourishing life. These make up the acronym 'PERMA' and are: Positive emotion, Engagement, Relationships, Meaning, Accomplishment.

> ### ⚙ Activity: Reflection
>
> In your work and in your wider life, what events, activities, thoughts or feelings make you feel good? What is important to you, in work and in life? What are you trying to achieve?

We will look at ways to improve wellbeing below, but first let us consider the contribution of positive psychology to understanding health.

Positive Psychology and Health

A comprehensive review (Steptoe et al., 2015) of the relationship between wellbeing, health and ageing concludes that there is a two-way relation between physical health and wellbeing. That is, poor health leads to reduced wellbeing, while high wellbeing can reduce physical health impairments. There was also evidence that better wellbeing is associated with surviving longer. So, understanding wellbeing and how to promote it is important. Many constituents of wellbeing have been studied from a positive psychology perspective; three of the most comprehensively appraised are '**sense of coherence**', '**optimism**' and 'benefit-finding and **posttraumatic growth**' (Aspinwall and Tedeschi, 2010).

Sense of coherence: is defined as *'an individual's global view of life, based on how comprehensible, manageable and meaningful life appears to them'* (Rohani et al., 2010: 2797). The term arises originally from the work of sociologist Aaron Antonovsky (1987) who proposed that an adverse event, such as work stress or illness, will be less stressful if the person experiencing it can understand it and feels they have the resources to manage it (note the link with **self-efficacy**) as this will lead to a sense that the event is tolerable. A sense that life is meaningful in some sense is what is thought to drive people to understand and manage adverse events (Aspinwall and Tedeschi, 2010).

A systematic review (Eriksson and Lindstrom, 2006) found 458 scientific publications and 13 doctoral theses that examine the relationship between sense of coherence and health. There was strong evidence that sense of coherence is health promoting, especially for mental health, that it strengthens resilience and helps develop a positive subjective state of health. Findings were independent of participant age, sex, ethnicity, nationality or of study design.

Optimism: is a generalised tendency to expect good things to happen. In research, optimism has been considered by some researchers to be at one end of a scale where pessimism is at the other end, but others have considered optimism and pessimism to be separate constructs. Optimism has been treated as a dispositional trait or as an explanatory style; some have equated it with 'hope' (Sharpe et al., 2011). People scoring high on optimism measures have been found to report higher levels of quality of life and better physical and mental wellbeing than those with lower scores or than those scoring high on pessimism scales; optimism is associated with healthy lifestyles, better coping and adaptive cognitive responses such as psychological flexibility and problem solving (Conversano et al., 2010).

A systematic review of 83 studies examining the relationship between optimism and physical health (Rasmussen et al., 2009) found effect sizes between -0.13 and 0.42 (mean 0.17), the variation is likely to be explained by the authors of the included studies having measured optimism in different ways. An association with optimism was found for both objective and subjective measure of health, although effect sizes were larger for the latter (Rasmussen et al., 2009). Warner and colleagues (2012) conducted a longitudinal study of 309 older adults (aged 65–85 years) with **multimorbidity** to determine whether the effect of objective physical functioning on subjective physical functioning is modified by health-specific optimism; they also considered self-efficacy as a **mediator**. They found that subjective ratings of physical functioning were predicted by both objective physical functioning and optimism but that optimism predicted subjective physical functioning only for those with low self-efficacy. The authors suggest that optimistic people may underestimate their vulnerability but at the same time overestimate their ability to cope (self-efficacy).

Benefit-finding and posttraumatic growth: Finding benefit in the presence of adversity is associated with less depression and better wellbeing (Helgeson et al., 2006) and was discussed in Chapter 3 in relation to positive **illness perceptions**. Posttraumatic growth, also known as stress-related growth, is a related concept. It refers to the experience of personal growth while dealing with stress and trauma, including diagnosis of physical illness (Aspinwall and Tedeschi, 2010). The trauma may cause an individual to reappraise their world view; personal growth occurs when this leads to changes such as a greater sense of personal strength, appreciation of life, improved relationships, spiritual change, new life opportunities or positive behaviour changes (Aspinwall and Tedeschi, 2010).

Barskova and Oesterreich (2009) reviewed the literature around posttraumatic growth following illness diagnosis. They found studies in cancer, HIV/AIDS, cardiac disease, multiple sclerosis and rheumatoid arthritis. Factors found to be associated consistently with posttraumatic growth included quality of **social support**, coping strategies and various indicators of mental and physical health.

So far, we have reviewed how researchers have defined the concept of wellbeing and some of the constructs that have been found to be associated with it. We have also explored the link between wellbeing and mental and physical health. Let us now consider what we might do to improve our own wellbeing and that of others.

IMPROVING WELLBEING

How to improve wellbeing is the subject of numerous popular psychology books and research articles and an aim of many psychological therapies. Here we will consider some current evidence-based approaches: Five Ways to Wellbeing, positive psychology interventions and **mindfulness**.

Five Ways to Wellbeing

The New Economics Foundation (NEF), an independent 'think-and-do tank', was commissioned by the UK Government to develop a set of evidence-based actions to improve personal wellbeing. Their report 'Five Ways to Wellbeing' (Aked et al., 2008) builds on a range of evidence, much of which arises from the positive psychology literature. The authors noted that much of the evidence was cross-sectional (so long-term effects could not be known) and that there is a lack of effect sizes (so we cannot tell how important each action is); in view of this they recommend an holistic approach to improving wellbeing.

The report identifies five actions demonstrated by research evidence to improve wellbeing. These are summarised as: connect, be active, take notice, keep learning, give. The full report can be accessed at: www.neweconomics.org/publications/entry/five-ways-to-wellbeing-the-evidence, and the five actions, as specified in the report, are reproduced in Box 6.2 below.

Box 6.2: Five Ways to Wellbeing (Aked et al., 2008)

Connect with the people around you. With family, friends, colleagues and neighbours. At home, work, school or in your local community. Think of these as the cornerstones of your life and invest time in developing them. Building these connections will support and enrich you every day.

Be active. Go for a walk or run. Step outside. Cycle. Play a game. Garden. Dance. Exercising makes you feel good. Most importantly, discover a physical activity you enjoy and that suits your level of mobility and fitness.

Take notice. Be curious. Catch sight of the beautiful. Remark on the unusual. Notice the changing seasons. Savour the moment, whether you are walking to work, eating lunch or talking to friends. Be aware of the world around you and what you are feeling. Reflecting on your experiences will help you appreciate what matters to you.

Keep Learning. Try something new. Rediscover an old interest. Sign up for that course. Take on a different responsibility at work. Fix a bike. Learn to play an instrument or how to cook your favourite food. Set a challenge you will enjoy achieving. Learning new things will make you more confident as well as being fun.

Give. Do something nice for a friend, or a stranger. Thank someone. Smile. Volunteer your time. Join a community group. Look out, as well as in. Seeing yourself, and your happiness, linked to the wider community can be incredibly rewarding and creates connections with the people around you.

Positive Psychology Interventions

Positive psychology researchers have designed and tested a range of interventions to improve wellbeing. A systematic review (Bolier et al., 2013) of the effectiveness of positive psychology interventions for the general public and for people with specific psychosocial problems identified 39 studies (n=6,139). The authors conclude that positive psychology interventions are effective for improving both wellbeing (standardised mean difference for wellbeing = 0.34) and depressive symptoms (standardised mean difference for depressive symptoms = 0.23). Many examples of positive psychology interventions, which varied in intensity and delivery (e.g. group, individual, self-help), were reported in the included studies. To be included in the review, interventions had to be '*aimed at raising positive feelings, positive cognitions or positive behaviour as opposed to interventions aiming to reduce symptoms, problems or disorders*'. They also had to have been '*explicitly developed in line with the theoretical tradition of positive psychology*'.

Typical positive psychology interventions include: increasing a feeling of gratitude, noticing positive experiences and identifying and using strengths (i.e. character strengths or talents) in a new way. Box 6.3 details some examples of positive psychology interventions which have been found to improve wellbeing, at least in some people. It is not known yet which are most effective in which people (are some inappropriate for some cultures or personality types perhaps?), how often they should be carried out to have lasting effects or whether, and under what condition, they may have detrimental effects.

Box 6.3: Positive psychology interventions – examples

Gratitude interventions:

1. Keep a gratitude journal – each week, write down five things that you have been grateful for that week. There may be little change each week as some things, such as 'good friends', 'supportive family', 'good health', will be ongoing. Nevertheless, it is the prompt to focus on these things that improves wellbeing, and some things may be more salient in a particular week (e.g. supportive friends following a crisis).

(Continued)

(Continued)

2. Write a 'thank you' letter to someone who has helped you (known as a gratitude letter), and deliver that letter to them (known as a gratitude visit).

Positive experience interventions:

1. Each night, write down, or bring to mind, three positive things that have happened during the day.
2. Remember a positive experience or event and replay it in your mind, focus on every detail and pay attention to the associated positive emotions and thoughts.

Strengths interventions:

1. Take a strengths test (for instance, Seligman's VIA strengths survey: www.viacharacter.org) or ask someone who knows you well to identify your strengths and plan a way to use one or more of your strengths differently. The idea is that developing your strengths will be intrinsically satisfying.
2. Strengths include qualities such as perseverance, modesty, kindness, creativity, curiosity, humour, openness, etc.

    i. If you chose perseverance, you could set yourself a difficult task (e.g. performing an exercise regimen, building a model, completing a puzzle). Notice how the act of perseverance makes you feel and what thoughts are associated with it.
    ii. If you chose curiosity, you could go somewhere you have not been before or identify and carry out a new activity. When in the new place or carrying out the activity, take notice of everything (sights, sounds, smells, sensations, tastes) that is new to you. Notice how they make you feel and what thoughts you have about them.

⚙ Activity: Reflection

Which of the five ways to wellbeing or positive psychology interventions in Box 6.3 could you try? Pick one and try setting yourself a SMART goal to achieve it.

Mindfulness

Mindfulness is more of an **attitude** to life than a wellbeing intervention. It is about living consciously in the present rather than worrying about the future or dwelling in the past. Wellbeing interventions, such as Five Ways to Wellbeing and some positive psychology interventions, assume that people feel better if they have more positive than negative experiences. In contrast, being mindful means experiencing life as it is, without judgement, and accepting ourselves and others as we are, with **compassion**. The aim of mindfulness is to increase our awareness both of the world around us and within us. It teaches us to notice our thoughts and emotions before we get caught up in them and overtaken by them. The following quote sums up what mindfulness teaches:

> When unhappiness or stress hover overhead, rather than taking it all personally, you learn to treat them as if they were black clouds in the sky, and to observe them with friendly curiosity as they drift past. (Williams and Penman, 2011: 5)

Mindfulness is informed by ancient Buddhist meditation practices. In the 1970s, student of Buddhism and Professor of Medicine, Jon Kabat-Zinn combined both disciplines to develop a secular training in mindfulness called mindfulness-based stress reduction (MBSR; see Box 6.4). This has been found to be helpful for health professionals in managing stress, reducing burnout, and improving well-being and quality of life (Cohen-Katz et al., 2005; Shapiro et al., 2005; Irving et al., 2009). The practice of mindfulness has been found to be associated with changes in grey matter concentration in brain regions that regulate emotion, self-referential processing and learning and memory (Hölzel et al., 2011) and with improved immune functioning (Hoffman et al., 2012; Lengacher et al., 2012; Carlson et al., 2013).

Box 6.4: Mindfulness-based stress reduction (MBSR)

- MBSR is an eight-week programme comprising one two-hour class per week plus a one-day retreat
- Participants are expected to complete a mindfulness-based meditation daily for about 45 minutes. This is intended to become a daily habit continued after the course
- Material covered includes dealing with stress, pain, depression, anxiety or disease
- Practical exercises include yoga, meditation and 'the body scan'
- The body scan is designed to increase body awareness and involves focusing on each part of the body, slowly moving from the toes to the top of the head. Guided recordings are freely available on the internet for beginners

Mindfulness techniques also have been combined with cognitive behavioural therapy (CBT) to develop psychological treatments, such as mindfulness-based cognitive therapy (MBCT) (Segal et al., 2001) and acceptance and commitment therapy (ACT) (Hayes, 2004). These therapies are classed as 'third wave CBT therapies' because they build on behaviour change therapies (first wave) and **cognition** changing therapies (second wave; see Box 6.5). Third wave therapies have been found to be effective for treating common mental disorders (Hofmann et al., 2010; Churchill et al., 2013).

Box 6.5: Third wave CBT therapies

In classical CBT, the client is taught to reappraise the triggers of emotional responses and to change the *content* of thoughts (e.g. replacing a catastrophic interpretation of a difficult situation with one that is more balanced, see Chapter 2).

Third wave cognitive behavioural therapies teach people instead to change the *function* of their cognitions. Unhelpful functions include:

- 'thought suppression' where the person is consciously trying to force distressing thoughts out of their minds
- 'experiential avoidance' where the person tries hard not to experience negative thoughts, emotions or bodily sensations (e.g. having an alcoholic drink to calm yourself).

These unhelpful functions are addressed using techniques such as:

Mindfulness – to increase conscious awareness and the ability to observe thoughts as private, fleeting mental events with which the individual can choose to engage or not to engage.

Acceptance – to embrace unwanted thoughts and feelings.

Cognitive defusion – to let go of strongly held beliefs which are preventing the client from living the life they want.

CHAPTER SUMMARY

Work stress and burn out were considered in relation to the work of healthcare professionals. Work stressors and other risks to health inherent in nursing and related work were identified.

The importance of nurse, midwife and health visitor health to their patients and their employers as well as to themselves was highlighted.

How psychologists have operationalised the term 'wellbeing' and the constructs of which it is considered to comprise were discussed. These were: life evaluation, hedonic wellbeing and eudemonic wellbeing.

The link between wellbeing and health was demonstrated. The relationship between health, the positive psychology constructs of 'sense of coherence', 'optimism' and 'benefit-finding and posttraumatic growth' appraised.

Approaches to improving wellbeing were detailed and reviewed. These were: Five Ways to Wellbeing, positive psychology interventions and mindfulness.

CONSOLIDATE YOUR LEARNING

 Activity: Quiz

(Answers can be found at the end of this book.)

1. List some nursing-related stressors which have been identified through research.
2. The construct of 'wellbeing' has been defined in terms of three broad dimensions (Steptoe et al., 2015): life satisfaction, hedonic wellbeing and eudemonic wellbeing. Briefly define each dimension.
3. It has been proposed that a stressful life event will be tolerated better if the person experiencing it has the sense that life is comprehensible, manageable and meaningful. How have psychologists labelled this sense?
4. List the 'five ways to wellbeing' (Aked et al., 2008).

⚙ **Activity: Reflection**

Looking after yourself is important for you, your family, your patients and wider society.

- How good is your wellbeing?
- Test your eudemonic and hedonic wellbeing using the Warwick-Edinburgh Wellbeing Scale: www2.warwick.ac.uk/fac/med/research/platform/wemwbs
- On which items was your score low?
- What could you do to feel better?
- Are there ideas in this book which could help?
- Think about your patients. Is there anyone whose wellbeing you would consider especially low?
- How could you help them to incorporate some of the 'five ways to wellbeing' in their life?
- What behaviour change approaches could you use to help them succeed?

FURTHER READING

Positive psychology – an easy to read introduction from the 'Father' of positive psychology: Seligman, M.E.P. and Csikszentmihalyi, M. (2000) Positive psychology: an introduction. *American Psychologist.* 55(1): 5–14.

Mindfulness – this popular book is an eight-week course which includes a CD of guided meditations: Williams, M. and Penman, D. (2011) *Mindfulness: A Practical Guide to Finding Peace in a Frantic World.* London: Piatkus.

USEFUL WEBSITES

Wellbeing resources and information: The What Works Centre for Wellbeing has compiled a useful set of links around wellbeing. http://whatworkswellbeing.org/wellbeing-2/links/

Nursing Standard's 'Eat well, nurse well' campaign. http://journals.rcni.com/page/ns/campaigns/eat-well-nurse-well

Numerous websites provide information and resources on mindfulness and on managing psychological distress, see: http://bemindful.co.uk/ and www.getselfhelp.co.uk/

Apps for phones or tablets can be used for mindfulness on the go! For example see: https://www.headspace.com/headspace-meditation-app

7 PUTTING IT ALL TOGETHER

Key Learning Objectives

At the end of this chapter you will be able to explain:

- How the health psychology topics you have learnt from this book relate to each stage in the life-course
- The competencies needed by nurses, midwives and health visitors to practise in a psychologically-informed manner
- How to apply your health psychology knowledge to your practice

INTRODUCTION

Whatever their specialist field, nurses, midwives and health visitors are helping patients and their families at each stage of life to manage illness and to stay as well as they can be. Throughout this book we have considered how knowledge of **health psychology** can help us to do this in the most effective and evidence-based way.

In Chapters 2, 3 and 4 of this book, we focused on the application of health psychology to managing emotions and their impact on health, to improving self-management of long-term conditions and to promoting healthy choices. Case examples describing patients from different age groups and relevant to the range of fields of nursing were provided. However, at each stage of the life-course specific issues are likely to arise in relation to emotions, self-management and health living. In this final chapter, we will highlight some of the key life-stage-related issues which may need to be considered when applying health psychology theory and techniques. You will be directed to the relevant sections of this book to help refresh your memory.

Whatever the life-stage of our patients and in whatever field we are practising as nurses, midwives and health visitors, we must adhere to the professional standards of practice and behaviour expected by our professional bodies at both pre- and at post-registration. This includes ensuring that we have the appropriate competencies to practice. In this chapter, we will consider the competencies required to practise in a health psychology-informed manner. Let us start by thinking about health psychology across the life-course.

HEALTH PSYCHOLOGY ACROSS THE LIFE-COURSE

Having read this book, you will be very aware of the impact of thoughts, feelings and behaviours on your patients' wellbeing and disease outcomes and on how they respond to and manage illness and its prevention. People's thoughts, feelings and behaviours vary according to their life-stage and its associated health-related issues and challenges.

Below we highlight some key health-related issues associated with each life-stage (other than adulthood which is well covered in earlier chapters and on which the majority of health psychology research has focused), suggest some potentially useful health psychology interventions and draw your attention to relevant sections of this book. Awareness of these issues will be useful when applying health psychology theories and techniques to help patients to cope with troublesome emotion, to manage their long-term conditions and to make healthy choices. Some case examples are provided which show how knowledge of health psychology can help health professionals to provide improved care.

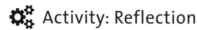 Activity: Reflection

As you read each life-course-related section, consider:

- Individual patients or people you know who are at this stage in life – what kind of problems are you aware that they have encountered? (They may be different to the ones covered here.)
- The possible health beliefs or illness perceptions which may be associated with the highlighted issues – what could you do to address unhelpful ways of thinking?
- The barriers to self-management or to making healthy choices that may occur at a particular life-stage – how could you help a patient facing one of these barriers?

Conception

Working with those who are planning to conceive may be routine for midwives and health visitors, but nurses working across a range of settings will also come into contact with such people. These may be patients receiving treatment for infertility or other, unrelated conditions, or they may be relatives or carers of your patients.

Emotions and Health

Psychological distress is commonly associated with miscarriage (Lok and Neugebauer, 2007), abortion (Bellieni and Buonocore, 2013) and infertility treatment (Rockliff et al., 2014). Nurses, midwives and health visitors will need excellent communication skills and the ability to determine whether psychological distress will resolve naturally or is at a level that requires intervention (see Chapter 2: Detecting Common Mental Disorders, p. 32).

Improving Self-management

People are much more likely to conceive if they are healthy, so optimal management of long-term conditions is important in people who are planning a family. This will include adherence to appropriate medications. Understanding of illness perceptions around medications adherence will be important for health professionals caring for these patients (see Chapter 3: Treatment Adherence, p. 52).

Promoting Healthy Choices

Being healthy by stopping smoking, reducing alcohol intake and by being a healthy weight is important for conception. Being overweight can reduce the chances of conception since fat cells produce oestrogen, too much of which prevents ovulation. Women who are underweight may also have trouble conceiving due to insufficient oestrogen for ovulation to occur. Almost any of the behaviour change techniques mentioned in this book may be applied to help people improve their smoking, diet and exercise choices. Using principles from motivational interviewing (MI) (Miller and Rollnick, 1991) may be a particularly practical approach (see Chapter 4: Motivational Interviewing (MI), p. 80).

Nurses, midwives and health visitors may also be involved in supporting contraceptive use in women who do not want to become pregnant. A systematic review of RCTs (Warriner, 2012) that tested a theoretical approach to improving contraceptive use found a lack of evidence to determine which approaches work best. Until more evidence is produced, nurses, midwives and health visitors will need to rely on their clinical judgement and knowledge of the individual when working with such patients. For instance, in women who are ambivalent about becoming pregnant, motivational interviewing can be used to explore that ambivalence in relation to their contraceptive use (Petersen et al., 2004); this is illustrated in the case example.

 ## Case Example: Motivational interviewing and contraceptive use

Jane is a sexual health nurse. Talitha is 25 years old and has arrived in clinic for her first cervical smear test. She is in a regular relationship, and though she and her partner do not currently live together, Talitha feels that they will move in together once they have decided to start a family. In the meantime, she is taking the combined oral contraceptive pill.

Jane questions Talitha about her contraceptive use and learns that, despite her assertion that she wants to avoid pregnancy, her pill-taking behaviour is rather erratic. Talitha reports several 'near misses' where she has thought she might be pregnant when she did not want to be due to having missed several doses.

Jane has established a good rapport with Talitha and decides to explore her behaviour using motivational interviewing techniques. Jane senses that Talitha is actually

(Continued)

(Continued)

ambivalent around becoming pregnant. Jane gently explores this ambivalence with her. They discuss what would be good about becoming pregnant now – Talitha feels her partner would move in with her sooner. They discuss the disadvantages of an unplanned pregnancy – Talitha recognises that it could 'put a strain' on her relationship with her partner who is clear that he is 'not ready to be a dad'; having a baby would also put financial pressures on the couple.

Talitha feels that on balance she doesn't really want to be pregnant yet, though might want to be soon. The discussion with Jane has highlighted for Talitha a discrepancy between her pill-taking behaviour and her goal of not becoming pregnant. Talitha starts to become defensive saying she is too busy to remember her pills and that her partner does not like to wear condoms. Jane suggests that other types of contraception such as an IUD or a contraceptive injection might be easier for her to manage.

Jane and Talitha discuss the advantages and disadvantages of each method. Talitha opts for the contraceptive injection, which will protect her against pregnancy for the next 12 weeks when she and her partner can reassess their situation.

Pregnancy

Emotions and Health

Pregnancy can be a source of stress for some women and their partners. This may be especially the case where a pregnancy is unplanned or unwanted. The women or couple may seek the help of nurses, midwives and health visitors in deciding whether to continue or discontinue the pregnancy. However, even wanted pregnancies can be stressful due to impacts on employment, finances, relationships, physical wellbeing and general uncertainty about the future. The ability to detect clinically important distress (see Chapter 2: Detecting Common Mental Disorders, p. 32) and to help patients manage stress (see Chapter 2: Stress, p. 21, and Chapter 6: Improving Wellbeing, p. 120) will be useful for nurses, midwives and health visitors working with pregnant women and their families.

Improving Self-management

In pregnant women with LTCs optimal self-management is important to reduce the impact of the condition on the foetus. A full medications review will be needed to ensure that prescribed medications are safe in pregnancy, and, for some, discontinuation or adjustment of medication can make management of their condition and symptoms more complex. However, for most women it is important that usual care is continued. For instance, asthma is associated with a range of adverse maternal and perinatal outcomes, but there is strong evidence that improved asthma control can improve health outcomes (Bain et al., 2014). Erroneous illness perceptions concerning medication use in pregnancy may hinder self-management; the information in Chapter 3: The Role of Illness Perceptions in Non-adherence will be useful to nurses, midwives and health visitors working with women who need to take regular medication during pregnancy (p. 52).

Many pregnant women will also have to cope with unpleasant symptoms such as nausea and back ache. The information in Chapter 5: Managing Enduring Physical Symptoms will help nurses, midwives and health visitors working with such women; the principles in the section on **chronic** pain (p. 89) may be especially applicable.

Promoting Healthy Choices

Both being underweight and obesity are risk factors for miscarriage (Feodor Nilsson et al., 2014). Being overweight is a risk factor for **gestational diabetes,** which is associated with adverse outcomes for the mother and baby. Alcohol misuse is associated with **foetal alcohol syndrome** and tobacco smoking during pregnancy is associated with pregnancy complications, stillbirth, low birthweight and preterm birth and long-term implications for women and babies (Chamberlain et al., 2013).

Pregnant women may therefore need support to lose weight, exercise more, eat healthily, reduce their alcohol use and to stop smoking. Nurses, midwives and health visitors may also need to help pregnant women adhere to recommended vitamin or mineral supplements and to avoid certain foods (recommendations as to which may vary between countries and healthcare systems). A range of interventions may be needed (See Chapter 4: Promoting Healthy Choices).

Labour, Birth and the Post-natal Period

Emotions and Health

Social support during pregnancy is important for the health of mothers and babies (Hodnett et al., 2010), and continuous support during labour is also beneficial (Hodnett et al., 2013). The role of social support in reducing stress is explained in Chapter 2, p. 31. Healthcare professionals can help women identify sources of social support as part of coping planning for labour (see Chapter 4: Action Planning and Coping Planning, p. 73). In addition, the post-natal period is well known to be associated with depression. Healthcare professionals in contact with these women should be aware of the potential risk factors and methods of screening. See Chapter 2: Box 2.4: Detecting CMDs – 'Women in the perinatal period' to remind yourself of these.

Improving Self-management

Women who have just given birth may be at risk of neglecting their own health due to the pressures of caring for a newborn (and very often the demanding siblings of the new arrival!), so may need additional support to manage existing conditions. Some drugs may be contraindicated when breast feeding, or erroneous illness perceptions may interfere with medications adherence as discussed in the section on pregnancy above (see Chapter 3: The Role of Illness Perceptions in Non-adherence, p. 55).

Promoting Healthy Choices

Eating a healthy, balanced diet is especially important when breast feeding. In some countries, breast feeding mothers are also encouraged to take vitamin D supplements. Techniques such as goal setting and action planning (see Chapter 4: Goals, p. 72) may be useful to help new mothers to ensure that they make time in their busy schedules to prepare and eat regular, healthy meals and to take supplements.

Childhood

Emotions and Health

About half of all lifetime cases of mental illness may start by age 14 years, though there may be years between the first onset of symptoms and the seeking or receipt of treatment (Kessler et al., 2005b). Estimates vary, but research suggests that 20 per cent of children have a mental health problem in any given year and about 10 per cent at any one time (St John et al., 2005). Nurses, midwives and health visitors working with children and their families should be aware of potential risk factors and how to recognise mental health problems in children (see Chapter 2: Box 2.4: Detecting CMDs – 'Children and young people').

Improving Self-management

Each developmental stage of childhood is associated with different issues and challenges for children with health conditions and for parents managing their child's long-term condition. For instance, in the period between childhood and adolescence conflict between child and parent expectations may start to arise. A systematic evaluation of self-management support interventions for children and young people with long-term conditions (Kirk et al., 2013) highlighted a lack of evidence for the effectiveness of such interventions, though there was some evidence suggesting that the most promising interventions target both children/young people and parents, use group methods and/or e-health interventions. This should be considered when applying to children and young people information on self-management support provided in Chapter 3.

Promoting Healthy Choices

Childhood obesity is a rising problem worldwide not least because obese children are more likely to become obese adults (Freedman et al., 2005) who have poor health outcomes and associated increased healthcare costs. In addition, overweight or obese children report lower levels of self-esteem and are at risk of bullying at school (Anesbury and Tiggemann, 2000). Targeting parental feeding habits has been found to be an effective intervention for improving healthy eating in children (McGowan et al., 2013); this is illustrated in the case example. The role of habits in health behaviour is discussed in Chapter 4: Box 4.7: The role of habit in behaviour change (p. 76).

 ## Case Example: Healthy eating in a two year old

When Fiona brought her two-year-old toddler Sam to Deborah's health visiting clinic, Deborah noticed that Sam was overweight. Deborah asked Fiona about Sam's diet and discovered that Sam was eating few fruits and vegetables. Fiona stated that neither she nor her partner Glenn were very keen on such food, though they were both aware that they needed to eat them to be healthy.

Deborah discussed further the importance of healthy eating, for both Sam and his parents, with Fiona. Fiona had not realised that overweight children were more likely to become overweight adults with ensuing health problems. By providing her with this evidence-based information, Deborah helped increase Fiona's **motivation** to improve the family's diet. Deborah provided Fiona with written information to take away to help keep up her motivation.

Deborah discussed barriers to healthy eating with Fiona. The main barrier that Fiona identified was cost. Deborah helped Fiona think about sources of fruit and vegetables that were cheaper than the local supermarket. Fiona realised that prices were likely to be cheaper at the local market and that she could easily drop past on her way home from dropping Sam at playgroup.

Having addressed this barrier, Deborah explained to Fiona how activities are easier to perform with repetition, that is, that building habits around healthy eating would make her and the family more likely to succeed. Between them, Deborah and Fiona agreed to start with a simple goal of each member of the family always eating one piece of fruit at breakfast. Once this behaviour had become automatic, further goals could be set to incorporate more fruit and vegetables into the family's diet.

Adolescence
Emotions and Health

As every parent knows, and (probably) as we all remember, adolescence is normally a time of high emotion. It can be difficult to determine what a normal level of emotion is and when troublesome emotions are a sign of something more serious which might require intervention. Mental health problems most likely to occur in adolescence include **self-harm**, substance abuse disorders, behaviour disorders, eating disorders and disorders relating to body image. However, depression is the most prevalent disorder among adolescents, though only about 25 per cent receive treatment (Garber et al., 2009). In addition, health professionals should be aware that subthreshold depression, depressive symptoms just below the diagnostic threshold for major depressive disorder, is common in adolescence, may be a precursor to major depressive disorder and is also associated with poor health outcomes (Garber et al., 2009; Wesselhoeft et al., 2013).

Improving Self-management

Self-management of long-term conditions such as diabetes, asthma and cystic fibrosis during adolescence is complex as responsibility for self-care transfers from parents to the young person, and because of the influence of peers (see case example: 'Adolescent with type 1 diabetes'). For instance, reports of diabetes-related conflict with parents have been found to be significant predictors of poor glycemic control in adolescents (Lancaster et al., 2015), and peer relationships during hospitalisation helped adolescents with cystic fibrosis 'begin to integrate their CF-related life experiences with their respective personal identities' (D'Auria et al., 2000). Nurses supporting adolescents and their parents to manage long-term conditions will need to be sensitive to these issues.

 ## Case Example: Adolescent with type 1 diabetes

Taylor is 14 years old and has had type 1 diabetes for one year and, up to now, has been managing well. Lately she has been feeling angry and resentful about having the disease, she feels that 'life is unfair' and that she has 'too much to cope with'. Her glucose levels remain well controlled, but her mother and the diabetes team are worried that her self-management may go downhill if she continues to feel this way.

Sheila, the diabetes nurse specialist, asks Taylor if anything has happened which has changed her **attitude** to her diabetes. It eventually becomes clear that Taylor has become more self-conscious about having diabetes; she does not want other people to know that she is diabetic and particularly resents wearing a medical identification tag. Sheila recognises self-consciousness as a common barrier to self-management in people Taylor's age; instead of trying to persuade Taylor to wear her usual tag (which is unlikely to work), Sheila tries to think of ways to help reduce Taylor's self-consciousness. She knows other teenagers who wear identification tags on their shoe instead of as a necklace or wrist-band and suggests this to Taylor who agrees to consider this option.

Sheila also knows that peer support is effective for improving self-management in adolescents with long term conditions (LTCs) – peers with similar issues may act as positive role models, share coping strategies and provide emotional support. She tells Taylor about a local group. Taylor is not ready to commit to that yet, but agrees to look at some websites especially for diabetic teenagers which Sheila tells her about. Sheila makes a plan to meet Taylor and follow up on these issues in a month's time. In the meantime, Taylor's mother agrees to look out for signs of deteriorating self-management and inform the diabetes team if necessary.

Promoting Healthy Choices

Eating healthily and exercising are important for adolescents as much as anyone else. This life-stage is where the individual will start to make their own choices and form habits which may be hard to break later. Issues relating to healthy living that may arise in adolescence include drug and tobacco use, alcohol misuse and sexual-risk behaviour. Knowledge of motivational interviewing and of how to build habits (see Chapter 4) may be particularly useful for nurses, midwives and health visitors working with adolescents.

Older Adulthood

Emotions and Health

As discussed in Chapter 2, mental health problems in later life may go untreated due to an assumption that they are a normal part of ageing. However, rates of depression are higher in older adulthood, perhaps because some of the risk factors for depression are more common, for instance being widowed/divorced, being a carer, loss of employment (including retirement), being socially isolated or lonely, or having poor physical health. According to a report by the Mental Health Foundation (see Useful Websites at the end of this chapter) neurobiological changes associated with getting older, prescribed medication and genetic susceptibility (which increases with age) are also risk factors for mental health problems. It is important for all health professionals working with older people to be aware of these risk factors and to ensure that older adults receive appropriate screening and help for mental health problems (see Chapter 2: Box 2.4: Detecting CMDs – special considerations (p. 34) and the case example below: 'Old age depression').

 ## Case Example: Old age depression

Alice is an 89-year-old widow who lives alone. She has poor mobility due to arthritis and has become increasingly housebound. It has been several weeks since she left her house. She has a daily visit from a carer, uses the meals on wheels service and her daughter visits daily to prepare a light supper. Lately, Alice has had regular visits from the community nursing team for management of leg ulcers related to mild heart failure and type 2 diabetes. Recently, several members of the team have noticed that Alice has been 'less chatty' than usual and has often been asleep when they arrive regardless of the time of day. The suppers made by her daughter are often left on the kitchen counter barely touched. Alice has always been a resilient person and when asked how she feels she replies 'a bit tired – that's all'.

On the whole, given her increasing frailty, the nurses are not surprised that Alice seems low. However, one nurse is aware that clinical depression can be overlooked

(Continued)

(Continued)

in the elderly. She administers the PHQ9 (Kroenke et al., 2001). A high score confirms the suspicions of the nurse who makes a referral to the local Improving Access to Psychological Therapies (IAPT) service. Following a full telephone assessment of her mental state, Alice is referred for a course of cognitive behavioural therapy for depression. Happily, where Alice lives this is available to be delivered by a specialist in old age depression who can make home visits.

Improving Self-management

A special consideration for health professionals working with older adults is that individuals are very likely to have more than one LTC. Little health psychology research has so far addressed the problem of **'multimorbidity'**, which is discussed in Chapter 3: Long-term Conditions (p. 43).

Promoting Healthy Choices

Health beliefs and health-related habits in older age are likely to have been held for a long time; this can make them harder to change. Some erroneous illness perceptions may have been held without negative effect, but now, in the context of age-associated health and lifestyle changes, may be detrimental. For instance, a belief that alcohol reduces stress may be harmless if alcohol consumption is low and confined to limited occasions. However, stress may increase in older age (for instance, due to illness, bereavement, financial pressures) and opportunities for drinking may be increased (for instance, more socialising and free time after retirement from work); this may lead to increased consumption (Britton and Bell, 2015). More alcohol consumption combined with increased physiological vulnerability to the effects of alcohol in older people (Wilkinson and Dare, 2014) may lead to serious health problems. Nurses can help older people to change their alcohol-related beliefs and drinking behaviour using motivational interviewing techniques (Miller and Rollnick, 1991) (see Chapter 4: Motivational Interviewing (MI), p. 80).

End of Life, Death and Bereavement

There is no agreed definition for the period referred to as 'end of life', which may also be referred to as 'terminal care', 'hospice care' and 'palliative care' with different implications in different settings (Izumi et al., 2012). Here we will use the term to refer to the period where patients need nursing care and where death within a few months would not be unexpected. Caring for patients in this period is clearly very complex – in the below section we highlight topics relevant to the content of this book; you are referred to Further Reading for more detailed information on nursing patients at the end of their lives.

Emotions and Health

The effects of grief, or adjustment to grief, on health are discussed in Chapter 2: Grief and Health (p. 25); nurses, midwives and health visitors should be alert to the risks to health for patients and carers following news of poor prognosis or bereavement.

With regard to dying patients themselves, health psychology research has been rather limited. It has however been recognised that clinical levels of depression or anxiety are not inevitable when a person knows they are dying. There is also some evidence that psychological interventions, especially those using CBT, improve depression even in patients with advanced cancer undergoing palliative care (Price and Hotopf, 2009). There are many settings in which end of life issues are faced regularly, including specialist palliative care, oncology, older persons' services and services for people with learning difficulties. Nurses, midwives and health visitors working in such settings, and those working with dying people in any setting, should be alert for signs of CMDs and arrange appropriate referral for psychological care.

When helping patients and their relatives to prepare for death, it will be useful for nurses to consider the individual's perception of a 'good death'. Qualitative research has shown that patients and families consider psychosocial and spiritual care as important as physical care (Steinhauser et al., 2000) and this should be considered when care planning.

Improving Self-management

The principles of self-management, which we learnt about in Chapter 3, will be relevant whether the patient is dying of cancer or another chronic illness. Self-management during the end of life phase is likely to involve treatment adherence (see Chapter 3: Treatment Adherence, p. 52), management of pain and other symptoms such as fatigue or treatment side effects such as nausea. Some such symptoms will be **acute** and managed by medications, though others will have been experienced by the patient for a long time. The information in Chapter 5: Managing Enduring Physical Symptoms will help health professionals working with patients with physical symptoms.

Shared decision-making (see Self-management, p. 45) will be particularly important to ensure that the patient receives care with which they are satisfied and with which they will engage. This may be in the context of 'advanced care planning' which may involve producing an 'advanced care directive' or 'living will' as a means of documenting preferences (Sanders et al., 2008). However, some patients used to managing long-term conditions find planning for death difficult so nurses should approach this carefully (Sanders et al., 2008).

Promoting Healthy Choices

Maintaining adequate hydration and nutrition are of particular concern in the end of life period for symptom control and quality of life. Patients may need support and advice to make healthy choices when their illness or its treatment affects their appetite or ability to eat and drink. However, poor nutritional care in the end of life period was highlighted among the failings of the Mid-Staffordshire Hospital (Francis, 2013) and in the controversy surrounding the use of the 'Liverpool Care Pathway for the Dying Patient' (Neuberger, 2013). A multidisciplinary approach along with clear, sensitive communication is recommended to support ethical decision-making and personalised, agreed nutritional goals which are reviewed and adapted regularly (Gillespie and Raftery, 2014).

Having reflected on the topics highlighted for different stages of the life-course, you may have identified other issues that you know have affected your patients. You should now be starting to be able to apply the health psychology knowledge you have gained from this book to those situations. However, to do this effectively in practice you will need to ensure you have the correct competencies and that you are working to appropriate professional standards; happily there are tools to help you with this, which we will detail. Let us start with describing what we mean by professional standards, before going on to explore the competencies you will need to work in a health psychology-informed manner.

NURSING, MIDWIFERY AND HEALTH VISITING PROFESSIONAL STANDARDS

Whether qualified or in training, nurses, midwives and health visitors, along with those working in other regulated professions, must adhere to the code of conduct set by their regulatory body. In the UK, our regulatory body is the Nursing and Midwifery Council (NMC). Codes of conduct present the professional standards to which individuals must adhere in order to be registered to practise. The principle aim of any code of conduct is to protect members of the public who come into contact with a member of the profession it addresses. The NMC Code of Conduct states that we should:

- Prioritise people
- Practise effectively
- Preserve safety
- Promote professionalism and trust

The Code is underpinned by professional standards for different activities or groups; for instance, standards for competence for registered nurse and midwives, standards for medications management, standards for pre-registration nursing-education and for midwifery-education. The NMC standards for competency are produced as a framework which identifies the knowledge, skills and attitudes nursing students must acquire by the end of their training programme before they are able to register to practise as nurses in the UK. The framework for pre-registration nurses comprises a set of competencies for each field of practice: adult, mental health, learning disabilities and children's nursing. Generic and field-specific competencies have been produced for four domains:

- Professional **values**
- Communication and interpersonal skills
- Nursing practice and decision-making
- Leadership, management and team working

Competence is defined by the Royal College of Nursing as: 'The state of having the knowledge, judgement, skills, energy, experience and motivation required to respond adequately to the demands of one's professional responsibilities' (Roach, 1992, cited in RCN, 2013: 2). Competency is relevant to all of the themes within the Code and to the standards underpinning it. In particular, the Code (NMC, 2015: 11) states that to protect patient and public safety you must: 'work within the limits of your competence, exercising your professional "duty of candour" and raising concerns immediately whenever you come across situations that put patients or public safety at risk. You take necessary action to deal with any concerns where appropriate'. If you wish to use health psychology-informed techniques in your practice, or encourage others to do so, you must therefore ensure that you, and they, are competent to do so. The recently developed 'framework for psychological interventions with people with persistent physical health conditions' (Roth and Pilling, 2015) is a useful guide and we will discuss this next.

COMPETENCIES FOR APPLYING HEALTH PSYCHOLOGY INTERVENTIONS

To qualify as a registered psychologist, it is necessary to have studied at doctoral level. The aim of this book is therefore not to turn nurses, midwives and health visitors into psychologists (and neither would anyone want to!), but to illustrate how theory and evidence from health psychology research can complement the specialist skills and knowledge that nurses, midwives and health visitors already possess. In the context of working with people with LTCs, which is a core aspect of many nurses' work, a competence framework for psychological interventions with people with persistent physical health conditions (Roth and Pilling, 2015) has been developed to ensure that psychology interventions are delivered effectively.

The Framework distinguishes between two ways of delivering psychological interventions by defining them as either 'formal psychological therapy' or 'psychologically-informed' (Roth and Pilling, 2015) which are so named as they employ strategies based on psychological principles. To deliver formal psychological therapy, one would be expected to have had in-depth training in order to have obtained the full range of competencies described in the Framework. However, fewer competencies are needed to deliver psychologically-informed interventions and these are well within the skill set of nurses, midwives and health visitors.

In setting out the competencies needed for delivering psychologically-informed interventions, the Framework (Roth and Pilling, 2015) distinguishes between skills and knowledge. Knowledge relevant to the practice setting and appropriate psychological theory is necessary for healthcare professionals to understand the rationale for applying their skills. It is this understanding of both how and why they are implementing an intervention that renders a professional 'competent'.

The Framework (Roth and Pilling, 2015) describes core professional competencies for work with people with physical health conditions and the related ethical and legal issues and professional skills and values. The competencies relating to ethical and legal issues include: knowledge of and ability to operate within professional and ethical guidelines; knowledge of and ability to work with issues of confidentiality and consent; knowledge of and ability to assess capacity. Competencies relating to professional skills and values include: ability to work with difference and ability to operate within and across organisations. These are professional competencies that every nurse, midwife and health visitor would be expected to have whether or not their work was psychologically-informed.

Competencies for applying psychologically-informed cross-condition interventions described by the Framework (Roth and Pilling, 2015) include: applying psychological principles in different service contexts (i.e. working with clinical services in medical settings and shared care in primary care) and applying psychological principles to support self-help or self-management (i.e. developing and implementing self-management programmes). Nurses, midwives and health visitors will be well used to working across settings and supporting patients' self-management.

Finally, core knowledge and clinical competencies around psychologically-informed interventions for people with persistent physical health conditions are defined (Roth and Pilling, 2015) as follows:

- Knowledge of a generic **model** of **medically unexplained syndromes** (MUS)
- Knowledge of presenting conditions
- Knowledge of the impact of physical health conditions in the context of life-stage
- Knowledge of generic models of adjustment of physical health conditions
- Promoting the client's capacity for adjustment
- Knowledge of models of behaviour change and strategies to achieve it
- Supporting clients' capacity for self-management

⚙ Activity: Reflection

Consider the knowledge and clinical competencies listed above. Do you feel confident that you possess all these competencies? If not, what could you do to improve? Try to identify the sections of this book which could inform you about each area of knowledge or skill. Use the identified sources of further reading at the end of each chapter to develop your understanding.

The competencies described were designed for working with people with persistent physical health conditions (including long-term conditions and medically unexplained syndromes), but are also relevant to working in a psychologically-informed manner with people with other conditions and when delivering interventions to promote healthy choices.

Some nurses, midwives and health visitors will have a more specific health promotion role than others, but all health professionals are expected to contribute through 'Making Every Contact Count (MECC)' (see p. 69). In Chapter 4: Behaviour

Change Interventions – Population Level (p. 84), we discussed briefly the use of health psychology in promoting public health. Public Health England, the public body established to promote health across the UK, has produced a tool to 'maximise nurses', midwives', health visitors' and allied health professionals' (AHPs') impact on improving health outcomes and reducing inequalities'. The tool is known as the 'Framework for Personalised Care and Population Health for Nurses, Midwives, Health Visitors and Allied Health Professionals (AHPs)' (PHE, 2014) (see Useful Websites at the end of this chapter). We consider this next.

NURSES, MIDWIVES AND HEALTH VISITORS AND HEALTH PROMOTION

The PHE Framework for Personalised Care and Population Health for Nurses, Midwives, Health Visitors and Allied Health Professionals (AHPs) (PHE, 2014) covers six key areas of population health activity: wider determinants of health; health improvement; health protection; healthcare public health; health, wellbeing and independence; and life-course. Healthcare professionals are shown how to use the tool through illustrated examples in each of these six activities. Examples are national health priorities and may change over time, but at the time of writing are: tuberculosis (health protection), antimicrobial resistance (health protection), falls (health, wellbeing and independence), beginning of life (life-course), healthy two year olds (life-course), respiratory disease (healthcare public health) and homelessness (wider determinants of health).

Health professionals can 'click' on each example to see relevant facts and information, national guidance, population level interventions, community level interventions, individual/family level interventions, outcome measures and examples of good practice. The interventions described have been judged to meet the criteria of:

1. Being evidence-based
2. Using appropriate technology
3. Promoting community participation in decisions about health services
4. Being provided at a cost the community can afford
5. Encouraging self-care and empowerment
6. Being the first line of contact with the health system
7. Bringing healthcare as close as possible to where people, live, work and play

---

⚙ **Activity**

Go to the PHE Framework for Personalised Care and Population Health for Nurses, Midwives, Health Visitors and AHPs website (www.gov.uk/government/publications/framework-for-personalised-care-and-population-health) and work through one of the examples relevant to your interests or area of practice.

The interventions in the PHE Framework are not described specifically as health psychology-informed, but many will be familiar to readers of this book who will bring additional skills and knowledge to their use of the Framework! The information in Box 7.1 is provided to help you remember key psychology-informed principles for health behaviour change which could be used with the PHE Framework. The outcomes linked to the PHE Framework include indicators from the Public Health Outcomes Framework, the NHS Outcomes Framework and the Adult Social Care Outcomes Framework, which represent nationally agreed outcomes and indicators to demonstrate improvements in health and social care.

Box 7.1: The EAST Framework – four simple ways to apply behavioural insights

The UK government's Behavioural Insights Team was set up to spread understanding of behavioural change across the policy community. They have developed a pragmatic, evidence-based framework to help people think about behaviour change. The Framework is based around four principles (which make up the acronym EAST: Easy, Attractive, Social, Timely), which are detailed in full in Service et al., 2014. A brief description from Service et al., 2014 (pages 4–6) is quoted here:

1. Make it Easy

    -   *Harness the power of defaults.* We have a strong tendency to go with the default or pre-set option, since it is easy to do so. Making an option the default makes it more likely to be adopted
    -   *Reduce the 'hassle factor' of taking up a service.* The effort required to perform an action often puts people off. Reducing the effort required can increase uptake or response rates
    -   *Simplify messages.* Making the message clear often results in a significant increase in response rates to communications. In particular, it's useful to identify how a complex goal can be broken down into simpler, easier actions

2. Make it Attractive

    -   *Attract attention.* We are more likely to do something that our attention is drawn towards. Ways of doing this include the use of images, colour or personalisation
    -   *Design rewards and sanctions for maximum effect.* Financial incentives are often highly effective, but alternative incentive designs – such as lotteries – also work well and often cost less

3. Make it Social

    -   *Show that most people perform the desired behaviour.* Describing what most people do in a particular situation encourages others to do the same. Similarly, policy makers should be wary of inadvertently reinforcing a problematic behaviour by emphasising its high prevalence
    -   *Use the power of networks.* We are embedded in a network of social relationships, and those we come into contact with shape our actions. Governments

can foster networks to enable collective action, provide mutual support, and encourage behaviours to spread peer-to-peer

- *Encourage people to make a commitment to others.* We often use commitment devices to voluntarily 'lock ourselves' into doing something in advance. The social nature of these commitments is often crucial

4. Make it Timely

- *Prompt people when they are likely to be most receptive.* The same offer made at different times can have drastically different levels of success. Behaviour is generally easier to change when habits are already disrupted, such as around major life events
- *Consider the immediate costs and benefits.* We are more influenced by costs and benefits that take effect immediately than those delivered later. Policy makers should consider whether the immediate costs or benefits can be adjusted (even slightly), given that they are so influential
- *Help people plan their response to events.* There is a substantial gap between intentions and actual behaviour. A proven solution is to prompt people to identify the barriers to action, and develop a specific plan to address them

Reproduced with permission of the Behavioural Insights Team

The EAST Framework (Service et al., 2014) is a useful aide memoire when thinking about delivering behaviour change at either the individual or population level. Throughout this book, health psychology theories have been described and critiqued to help you understand how or why health psychology interventions may work. On a more practical level, specific, evidence-based behaviour change techniques, such as 'ask, advise, act', feedback and monitoring, goal setting, action planning, coping planning, 'if, then rules', incentives and motivational interviewing, have been described, which can help when working with individuals to manage existing conditions and to make healthy choices. The Useful Websites section at the end of this chapter provides links to resources such as apps, work sheets and relaxation tools, which can facilitate this work. Above all, when working in a health psychology-informed manner to promote behaviour change, this book provides evidence to encourage you to: 1) use every opportunity, 2) offer support even when you are not sure the individual is interested, 3) use evidence-based behaviour change techniques and 4) review progress regularly. Finally, you are encouraged to take care of yourself, not only for your own sake and that of your families, but for your patients. Make use of the information and resources in this book to address unhelpful thoughts, manage troublesome emotions, cope with ill health, make healthy choices and improve your wellbeing.

CHAPTER SUMMARY

Life-stage-related issues to consider when working in a health psychology-informed manner have been highlighted.

The competencies needed to apply health psychology theories and techniques to nursing, midwifery and health visiting work have been described.

Key messages for effective behaviour change have been summarised.

You are reminded of the importance of your own wellbeing and encouraged to use your health psychology knowledge to take good care of yourself.

 Activity: Reflection

From what you have read here, have you been encouraged to work in a more health psychology-informed manner?

If so, how will you do this? If not, why not?

FURTHER READING

Psychology textbook for midwives: Raynor, M.D. (2010) *Psychology for Midwives: Pregnancy, Childbirth and Puerperium.* Milton Keynes: Open University Press.

Child and adolescent psychology textbook: Carr, A. (2006) *The Handbook of Child and Adolescent Clinical Psychology: A Contextual Approach.* London: Routledge.

Comprehensive text on all aspects of nursing people in the end of life phase: Nicol, J. and Nyatanga, B. (2014) *Palliative and End of Life Care in Nursing.* London: Sage.

Evidence, theory and values-based guide to planning health promotion: Green, J. and Tones, K. (2010) *Health Promotion: Planning and Strategies* (Second edition). London: Sage.

USEFUL WEBSITES

Report on mental health in older age by the Mental Health Foundation: www.mentalhealth. org.uk/help-information/mental-health-a-z/o/older-people/

An interactive map describing Roth and Pilling's (2015) competence framework for psychological interventions with people with persistent physical health conditions: www.ucl.ac. uk/clinical-psychology/competency-maps/physical-health-map.htm

PHE's Framework for Personalised Care and Population Health for Nurses, Midwives, Health Visitors and Allied Health Professionals (PHE, 2014): www.gov.uk/government/publications/framework-for-personalised-care-and-population-health

The NHS Choices Health Apps Library provides links to apps which have been reviewed by the NHS to ensure they are clinically safe and relevant to people living in England: http://apps.nhs.uk/

Self-help and therapist CBT-related tools to help individual behaviour change – includes worksheets for qualified therapists, but also simpler tools such as food diaries and activity planners as well as MP3 downloads: www.get.gg/

GLOSSARY

Acute   severe and sudden.

Angiogram   an X-ray test that uses dye to examine blood vessels.

Anxiogenic   causing anxiety.

Attention deficit hyperactivity disorder   a group of behavioural symptoms that include inattentiveness, hyperactivity and impulsiveness, often abbreviated to ADHD.

Attitude   a belief with a value component.

Autonomy   the perception of an individual that they are responsible for and have chosen their actions.

Avoidance behaviour   behaviour carried out with the intention of avoiding a stressful situation.

Behavioural contracts   verbal or written agreements between a healthcare professional and a patient intended to provide a record of agreed goals and actions.

Behavioural experiment   an activity designed to test whether someone's beliefs or behaviours are helpful or unhelpful.

Benefit finding   the perception that positive changes have occurred as a result of a traumatic or life-changing event.

Body mass index (BMI)   the relationship between an individual's weight and height, used as an index to determine whether they are at a healthy weight, i.e. a BMI of 20 to 25. It is calculated by dividing weight in kilograms by height in metres squared.

Brief interventions   short interventions that may involve discussion, negotiation or encouragement, provision of supportive materials and referral for further support.

Burnout   an extreme form of work stress, often associated with care-giving professions, that is characterised by emotional exhaustion, a sense of inefficacy and cynicism.

Chronic   persisting for a long time.

Chronic fatigue syndrome   an enduring condition characterised by extreme or unusual tiredness.

Circadian rhythms biological processes that follow an approximately 24-hour cycle, responding to light and other environmental triggers.

Cognition a thought process including beliefs and perceptions.

Compassion showing empathy and concern for another's, or one's own (self-compassion) welfare.

Compassion fatigue a condition, often associated with care-giving professions, that is characterised by a gradual depletion of compassion over time due to prolonged exposure to traumatic situations.

Confidence ruler a scale from 1 (not at all) to 10 (extremely confident) used to indicate a patient's confidence in achieving a goal.

Disability-adjusted life years (DALYs) a universal metric used to express the number of years lost due to ill-health, disability or early death across a given population.

Delphi-type study an interactive research method in which experts provide responses, for instance through a series of questionnaires, with the aim of evaluating accepted practices or assumptions and reaching a consensus of opinion.

Depressogenic causing depression.

Endometriosis a chronic condition in which womb tissue is found outside the womb within the pelvis.

Exposure subjection to something, normally through experience.

Fibromyalgia a medically unexplained syndrome characterised by widespread muscular or musculoskeletal pain.

Flourishing a positive psychology concept that defines the state of optimal wellbeing.

Foetal alcohol syndrome irreversible damage to a child's brain and growth due to exposure to alcohol during gestation.

Gestational diabetes a diabetic condition which develops in pregnancy (gestation); it is a risk factor for developing type 2 diabetes.

Guided discovery Socratic questioning in the context of cognitive behavioural therapy (CBT), whereby a therapist asks a client a series of questions designed to help them understand their current perception of a situation and to identify different ways of viewing it.

Health literacy the degree to which an individual has the ability to obtain, process and understand information in order to make appropriate health decisions.

Health promoting financial incentive intervention (HPFI) an intervention that involves a financial payment to encourage healthy behaviours.

Health psychology the study of psychological, social, biological and behavioural influences in health, illness and healthcare.

Illness perceptions an individual's beliefs about an illness or its management.

Implementation intention an internal strategy for instigating goal-directed behaviour in the presence of a contextual cue, often formed as an 'if, then rule'.

Intervention fidelity the degree to which the planned components of an intervention have been delivered as intended.

Mastery experience experience of success in a task which increases confidence in achievement or self-efficacy.

Mediator a variable which explains the relationship, for instance how or why it occurs, between two other variables.

Medically unexplained syndromes conditions that do not appear to have an identifiable organic cause or whose physiologicial mechanisms are poorly understood; for instance, irritable bowel syndrome, chronic fatigue syndrome and fibromyalgia.

Mindfulness a mental state defined by living consciously in the present.

Model a description of a process or system.

Moderator a variable which influences the strength or direction of a relationship between two other variables and so can tell you whether a relationship can or cannot be expected.

Motivation a reason for acting or behaving in a particular way.

Multimorbidity the concurrence of two or more chronic medical conditions in one person.

Myocardial infarction damage to the heart muscle caused by restricted blood flow, commonly known as a heart attack.

Non-malignant pain pain persisting beyond the time of expected healing which is not associated with progressively severe (malignant) disease.

Nudge a type of intervention that uses knowledge of human behaviour to guide someone in a desired direction.

Optimism a generalised tendency to expect or hope for a positive outcome.

Peer support assistance provided to patients or carers by people with a similar condition to the patient or with experience of caring for someone with a similar condition.

Positive psychology a branch of psychology that studies and aims to promote the positive aspects of human life such as happiness and wellbeing.

Posttraumatic growth positive change that occurs while dealing with stress and trauma. Also known as stress-related growth.

Psychopathology mental or behavioural disorder.

Resistance (in context of motivational interviewing) a refusal to accept or comply with a change that is deemed beneficial.

Revascularisation a medical procedure in which obstructed blood vessels are unblocked or surgically replaced to restore blood circulation to an organ or other part of the body.

Safety behaviour behaviour intended to protect against a fearful situation.

Self-control an individual's capacity to override dominant or habitual responses through self-regulatory behaviours.

Self-efficacy an individual's confidence in their ability to tolerate or successfully overcome a particular situation.

Self-harm the act of deliberate harm or infliction of injury to one's body commonly through cutting or burning.

Sense of coherence a worldview in which life appears comprehensible, manageable and meaningful.

Shared decision-making an approach to treatment whereby a patient and their healthcare professional make healthcare choices together, taking into account what is important to each person.

Sleep hygiene practices intended to foster better quality sleep on a regular basis.

Social capital the total amount of social resources available to an individual.

Social desirability bias the tendency to respond in a way that will be accepted by others.

Social network a network of people available to provide help and support.

Social norm   the expected behaviour in a particular situation.

Social support   help available from others within a social network.

Socratic questioning   a method of asking questions intended to stimulate discussion in order to improve understanding and to generate new ideas.

Somatic   relating to the body.

Subjective norm   an individual's perceived importance of a social norm.

Thinking error   an unhelpful belief or distorted way of thinking that contributes to troublesome emotion.

Value   a global, abstract guiding principle.

Very brief interventions   interventions that may take only a few seconds.

Wellbeing   a state of contented existence characterised by health and happiness and encompassing a range of psychological and social factors.

QUIZ ANSWERS

If you have trouble understanding, if words seem unfamiliar to you or if you need further explanation, check the glossary and reread the relevant sections in the book.

CHAPTER 1

1. The randomised controlled trial (RCT) is the best study design for determining the effectiveness of an intervention because of its ability to control for bias and for both known and unknown variables which may have an effect on outcomes above and beyond the intervention being tested.
2. A lack of evidence means that insufficient, good-quality trials have been conducted to determine whether or not an intervention works. A finding of evidence of no effect means that good-quality trials have found that an intervention did not work.
3. The HBM (Rosenstock, 1966; Becker, 1974) is a 'cognitive model' because it emphasises the role of beliefs in health behaviour.
4. 'Perceived behavioural control' is informed by 'internal control factors', such as perceived or known skills, abilities, feeling informed, and by 'external control factors', such as perceived or known obstacles, and opportunities.

CHAPTER 2

1. Symptoms of depression should have been present for at least two weeks in sufficient severity for most of every day for a diagnosis to be made.
2. There is some evidence that female gender, lower socioeconomic status, past history of CMD, alcohol misuse, antenatal and postnatal periods and medical illness are predictors of CMDs.
3. The relationship between CMDs and physical illness appears to be bidirectional (may go either or both ways). Biological mechanisms have been proposed, but behavioural factors are also predictors.
4. Thoughts, feelings, behaviour and physiology.

CHAPTER 3

1. Self-management is most effective when the patient is supported by clinicians and others, has high self-efficacy, has appropriate illness perceptions, adheres to their treatment regimen and when there is shared decision-making.

2. Illness perceptions impact on coping actions, emotional outcomes and self-management behaviour.
3. According to the 'Perceptions and Practicalities Model' (Horne, 2006), non-adherence can be considered as 'unintentional' or 'intentional', though, in a single patient, non-adherence may have both components.
4. According to the 'Necessity–Concerns Framework' (NCF) (Horne and Weinman, 1999), illness perceptions associated with treatment adherence can be classified as relating to either perceptions of the need for treatment or perceptions relating to concerns about potential adverse consequences.

CHAPTER 4

1. The NICE guidance on individual level behaviour change (NICE, 2014a) suggests that two groups of techniques – feedback and monitoring and goals and planning – are likely to be effective within interventions to change behaviours relating to alcohol, diet, physical activity and smoking.
2. SMART – specific, measurable, achievable, relevant, time-bound (though other texts may use slightly different words, the principles are the same).
3. OARS – open-ended questions, affirmation, reflective-listening, summarising. These are the four key skills needed to deliver motivational interviewing.
4. Interventions which nurses, midwives and health visitors can use to help with action planning and coping planning include: identifying barriers and facilitators, implementation intentions and behavioural contracts.

CHAPTER 5

1. The Fear-avoidance Model (Vlaeyen and Linton, 2000) has been used most comprehensively to explain health behaviours associated with enduring pain and fatigue.
2. Catastrophising. The cognitive behavioural model of panic (Clark, 1986) predicts a vicious cycle of catastrophic misinterpretation of the cause and/or consequences of symptoms leading to increasing fear and sympathetic arousal.
3. Sleep can be disrupted by: 1) sleep-interpreting processes – misperceptions, dysfunctional beliefs, expectations and attributions concerning sleep and the causes and consequences of poor sleep – and 2) sleep-interfering processes – cognitive, emotional and physiological arousal-producing processes that interfere with sleep such as anxiety, worry, pain or other symptoms.
4. People experiencing chronic fatigue commonly 'push themselves' or 'overdo things' during the times in which they are feeling better because they worry their fatigue will later prevent them from doing what they need or want to do. This tends to result in worse fatigue, followed by the need to rest more. Their sense of frustration is then increased further which leads to them 'overdoing things' again when they feel well.

CHAPTER 6

1. A factor analysis of studies using a range of measures of nursing-related stress (French et al., 2000) identified the following stressors: dealing with death and dying, conflict with physicians, inadequate preparation to deal with others' emotional needs, problems with peers, problems with supervisors, workload, uncertainty concerning treatment, dealing with patients and their families and feeling discriminated against (on the basis of age, gender and ethnicity).

2. In the study of wellbeing, life satisfaction refers to how people define the overall quality of their lives, hedonic wellbeing refers to experienced feelings or mood, eudemonic wellbeing refers to the person's judgement of the meaning and purpose of their life.

3. The sense that life is understandable and can be managed and is meaningful is known as a 'sense of coherence'.

4. The five ways to wellbeing are: connect, be active, take notice, keep learning, give (Aked et al., 2008).

REFERENCES

Abdel-Tawab, R., James, D.H., Fichtinger, A., Clatworthy, J., Horne, R. and Davies, G. (2011) Development and validation of the Medication-Related Consultation Framework (MRCF). *Patient Education and Counseling.* 83(3): 451–7.

Adriaanse, M.A., Vinkers, C.D.W., DeRidder, D.T.D., Hox, J.J. and DeWit, J.B.F. (2011) Do implementation intentions help to eat a health diet? A systematic review and meta-analysis of the empirical evidence. *Appetite.* 56: 183–93.

Ahlberg, K., Gaston-Johansson, F. and Mock, V. (2003) Assessment and management of cancer related fatigue in adults. *The Lancet.* 362: 640–50.

Ajzen, I. (1985) From intention to actions: a theory of planned behaviour, in J. Kuhl and J. Beckman (eds) *Action Control: From Cognition to Behaviour.* Heidelberg: Springer, pp. 11–39.

Ajzen, I. (1991) The Theory of Planned Behaviour. *Organizational Behavior and Human Decision Processes.* 50(2): 179–211.

Ajzen, I. and Madden, T.J. (1986) Prediction of global-directed behaviour: attitudes, intentions, and perceived behavioural control. *Journal of Experimental Social Psychology.* 22: 453–74.

Aked, J., Marks, N., Cordon, C. and Thompson, S. (2008) *Five Ways to Wellbeing: The Evidence.* London: New Economics Foundation. www.neweconomics.org/publications/entry/five-ways-to-well-being-the-evidence (accessed 1/12/15).

American Psychiatric Association. (2013) *Diagnostic and Statistical Manual of Mental Disorders* (Fifth edition). Washington, DC.

Andersson, M.A. and Conley, C.S. (2008) Expecting to heal through self-expression: a perceived control theory of writing and health. *Health Psychology Review.* 2: 138–62.

Anesbury, T. and Tiggemann, M. (2000) An attempt to reduce negative stereotyping of obesity in children by changing controllability beliefs. *Health Education Research.* 15(2): 145–52.

Antonovsky, A. (ed.) (1987) *Unraveling the Mystery of Health: How People Manage Stress and Stay Well.* San Francisco: Jossey-Bass.

Armitage, C.J. and Conner, M. (2001) Efficacy of the theory of planned behaviour: a meta-analytic review. *British Journal of Social Psychology.* 40: 471–99.

Armstrong, M.I., Birnie-Lefcovitch, S. and Ungar, M.T. (2005) Pathways between social support, family wellbeing, quality of parenting, and child resilience: what we know. *Journal of Child and Family Studies.* 14(2): 269–81.

Asnaani, A., Richey, J.A., Dimaite, R., Hinton, D.E. and Hofmann, S.G. (2010) A cross-ethnic comparison of lifetime prevalence rates of anxiety disorders. *Journal of Nervous and Mental Disease.* 198: 551–5.

Aspinwall, L.G. and Tedeschi, R.G. (2010) The value of positive psychology for health psychology: progress and pitfalls in examining the relation of positive phenomena to health. *Annals of Behavioural Medicine.* 39(1): 4–15.

Aveyard, P., Begh, R., Parsons, A. and West, R. (2012) Brief opportunistic smoking cessation interventions: a systematic review and meta-analysis to compare advice to quit and offer of assistance. *Addiction.* 107(6): 1066–73.

Bain, E., Pierides, K.L., Clifton, V.L., Hodyl, N.A., Stark, M.J., Crowther, C.A. and Middleton, P. (2014) Interventions for managing asthma in pregnancy. *Cochrane Database of Systematic Reviews*, Issue 10. Art. No.: CD010660. DOI: 10.1002/14651858.CD010660.pub2.

Bala, M.M., Strzeszynski, L., Topor-Madry, R. and Cahill, K. (2013) Mass media interventions for smoking cessation in adults. *Cochrane Database of Systematic Reviews*, Issue 6. Art. No.: CD004704. DOI: 10.1002/14651858.CD004704.pub3.

Bandura, A. (1977) *Self-efficacy: The Exercise Control*. New York: Freeman.

Bandura, A. (1986) *Social Foundations of Thought and Action*. Englewood Cliffs, NJ: Prentice Hall.

Barley, E.A., Walters, P., Tylee, A. and Murray, J. (2012a) General practitioners' and practice nurses' views and experience of managing depression in CHD: a qualitative interview study. *BMC Family Practice*. 13: 1.

Barley, E.A., Haddad, M., Simmonds, R., Fortune, Z., Walters, P., Murray, J., Rose, D. and Tylee, A. (2012b) The UPBEAT depression and CHD programme: using the UK Medical Research Council framework to design a nurse-led complex intervention for use in primary care. *BMC Family Practice*. 12(13): 119.

Barley, E.A., Walters, P., Haddad, M., Phillips, R., Achilla, E., McCrone, P., Van Marwijk, H., Mann, A. and Tylee, A. (2014) The UPBEAT nurse-delivered personalized care intervention for people with CHD who report current chest pain and depression: a randomised controlled feasibility trial. *PLOS ONE*. 9(6): e98704.

Barlow, J., Wright, C., Sheasby, J., Turner, A. and Hainsworth, J. (2002) Self-management approaches for people with chronic conditions: a review. *Patient Education and Counseling*. 48: 177–87.

Barnett, M. (2005) COPD: a phenomenological study of patients' experiences. *Journal of Clinical Nursing*. 14(7): 805–12.

Barth, J., Schumacher, M. and Herrmann-Lingen, C. (2004) Depression as a risk factor for mortality in patients with CHD: a meta-analysis. *Psychosomatic Medicine*. 66(6): 802–13.

Barskova T. and Oesterreich, R. (2009) Post-traumatic growth in people living with a serious medical condition and its relations to physical and mental health: a systematic review. *Disability and Rehabilitation*. 31(21): 1709–33.

Baumeister, R.F., Bratslavsky, E., Muraven, M. and Tice, D.M. (1998) Ego depletion: is the active self a limited resource? *Journal of Personality and Social Psychology*. 74: 1252–65.

Baumeister, R.F., Gailliot, M., DeWall, C.N. and Oaten, M. (2006) Self-regulation and personality: how interventions increase regulatory success, and how depletion moderates the effects of traits on behavior. *Journal of Personality*. 74: 1773–801.

Baumeister, R.F., Vohs, K.D. and Tice, D.M. (2007) The strength model of self-control. *Current Directions in Psychological Science*. 16: 351–5.

Bebbington, P.E. (1998) Epidemiology of obsessive-compulsive disorder. *British Journal of Psychiatry Supplement*. 35: 2–6.

Beck, A.T. (1967) *Depression: Clinical, Experimental, and Theoretical Aspects*. New York: Hoeber. Republished as *Depression: Causes and Treatment*. Philadelphia: University of Pennsylvania Press.

Beck, A.T., Ward, C.H., Mendelson, M., Mock, J. and Erbaugh, J. (1961) An inventory for measuring depression. *Archives of General Psychiatry*. 4: 561–71.

Becker, M.H. (ed.) (1974) *The Health Belief Model and Personal Health Behavior*. Thorofare, NJ: Charles B. Slack.

Belanger-Gravel, A., Godin, G. and Amireault, S. (2011) A meta-analytic review of the effect of implementation intentions on physical activity. *Health Psychology Review*. 7(1): 23–54.

Bellieni, C.V. and Buonocore, G. (2013) Abortion and subsequent mental health: review of the literature. *Psychiatry and Clinical Neurosciences*. 67(5): 310.

Benca, R.M. (2005) Diagnosis and treatment of chronic insomnia: a review. *Psychiatric Services.* 56: 332–43.

Benowitz, N.L. (2010) Nicotine addiction. *New England Journal of Medicine.* 362: 2295–303.

Benton, T., Staab, J. and Evans, D.L. (2007) Medical co-morbidity in depressive disorders. *Annals of Clinical Psychiatry.* 19(4): 289–303.

Berk, M., Williams, L.J., Jacka, F.N., O'Neil, A., Pasco, J.A., Moylan, S., Allen, N.B., Stuart, A.L., Hayley, A.C., Byrne, M. and Maes, M. (2013) So depression is an inflammatory disease, but where does the inflammation come from? *BMC Medicine.* 11: 200.

Berkman, N.D., Sheridan, S.L., Donahue, K.E., Halpern, D.J. and Crotty, K. (2011) Health literacy and health outcomes: an updated systematic review. *Annals of Internal Medicine.* 155(2): 97–107.

Berna, C., Tracey, I. and Holmes, E.A. (2012) How a better understanding of spontaneous mental imagery linked to pain could enhance imagery-based therapy in chronic pain. *Journal of Experimental Psychology.* 3(2): 258–73.

Bhugra, D. and Mastrogianni, A. (2004) Globalisation and mental disorders: overview with relation to depression. *British Journal of Psychiatry.* 184: 10–20.

BMA (2003) Investing in general practice: the new general medical services contract. BMA & NHS Employers.

Bodenheimer, T., Wagner, E.H. and Grumbach, K. (2002) Improving primary care for patients with chronic illness. *Journal of the American Medical Association.* 288(14): 1775–9.

Bodenheimer, T. and Handley, M.A. (2009) Goal-setting for behavior change in primary care: an exploration and status report. *Patient Education and Counseling.* 76: 174–80.

Bolier, L., Haverman, M., Westerhof, G.J., Riper, H., Smit, F. and Bohlmeijer, E. (2013) Positive psychology interventions: a meta-analysis of randomized controlled studies. *BMC Public Health.* 13: 119

Booker, L and Mullan, B. (2013) Using the temporal self-regulation theory to examine the influence of environmental cues on maintaining a healthy lifestyle. *British Journal of Health Psychology.* 18: 745–62.

Boorman, S. (2009) NHS Health and Wellbeing Review: DH. http://webarchive.national-archives.gov.uk/20130107105354/http:/www.dh.gov.uk/en/Publicationsandstatistics/Publications/PublicationsPolicyAndGuidance/DH_108799 (accessed 1/12/15).

Bootzin, R.R. and Epstein, D.R. (2011) Understanding and treating insomnia. *Annual Review of Clinical Psychology.* 7: 435–58.

Bosch-Capblanch, X., Abba, K., Prictor, M. and Garner, P. (2007) Contracts between patients and healthcare practitioners for improving patients' adherence to treatment, prevention and health promotion activities. *Cochrane Database of Systematic Reviews*, Issue 2. Art. No.: CD004808. DOI: 10.1002/14651858.CD004808.pub3.

Bradburn, N. (1969) *The Structure of Psychological Well-being.* Chicago: Aldine.

Breivik, H., Collett, B., Ventafridda, V., Cohen, R. and Gallacher, D. (2006) Survey of chronic pain in Europe: prevalence, impact on daily life, and treatment. *European Journal of Pain.* 10(4): 287–333.

Bridle, C., Riemsma, R.P., Pattenden, J., Sowden, A.J., Mather, L., Watt, I.S., Walker, A. (2005) Systematic review of the effectiveness of health behavior interventions based on the trans-theoretical model. *Psychology & Health.* 20(3): 283–301.

Britton, A. and Bell, S. (2015) Reasons why people change their alcohol consumption in later life: findings from the Whitehall II Cohort Study. *PLoS ONE.* 10(3): e0119421.

Broadbent, E., Petrie, K.J., Main, J. and Weinman, J. (2006) The brief illness perception questionnaire. *Journal of Psychosomatic Research.* 60 (6): 631–7.

Broman, J.E. and Lundh, L.G. (2003) Vicious cycles of sleeplessness: a new scale for insomnia. *Sleep.* 26: A298.

Burgess, M. and Chalder, T. (2009) *Overcoming Chronic Fatigue: A Self-help Guide Using Cognitive Behavioral Techniques.* London: Robinson.

Burnell, K., Charlesworth, G., Feast, A.R., Hoe, J., Poland, F.M. and Orrell, M. (2012) Peer support interventions for family carers of adults with chronic mental or physical illness who are living at home (Protocol). *Cochrane Database of Systematic Reviews,* Issue 11. Art. No.: CD010231. DOI: 10.1002/14651858.CD010231.

Burroughs, H.I., Lovell, K., Morley, M., Baldwin, R., Burns, A. and Chew-Graham, C. (2006) 'Justifiable depression': how primary care professionals and patients view late-life depression? A qualitative study. *Family Practice.* 23(3): 369–77.

Burnet, D., Plaut, A., Courtney, R. and Chin, M.H. (2002) A practical model for preventing type 2 diabetes in minority youth. *Diabetes Education.* 28(5): 779–95.

Burns, J.W., Quartana, P.J. and Bruehl, S. (2008) Anger inhibition and pain: conceptualizations, evidence and new directions. *Journal of Behavioural Medicine.* 31(3): 259–79.

Butler, C.C., Simpson, S.A., Hood, K., Cohen, D., Pickles, T., Spanou, C., McCambridge, J., Moore, L., Randell, E., Alam, M.F., Kinnersley, P., Edwards, A., Smith, C. and Rollnick, S. (2013) Training practitioners to deliver opportunistic multiple behaviour change counselling in primary care: a cluster randomised trial. *BMJ.* 346:f1191.

Cannon, W.B. (1932) *The Wisdom of the Body.* New York: Norton.

Carlson, L.E., Doll, R., Stephen, J., Faris, P., Tamagawa, R., Drysdale, E. and Speca, M. (2013) RCT of mindfulness-based cancer recovery versus supportive expressive group therapy for distressed survivors of breast cancer. *Journal of Clinical Oncology.* 31(25): 3119–26.

Carney, C.P., Jones, L. and Woolson, R.F. (2006) Detection and management of co-morbidity in patients with schizophrenia: a population based controlled study. *Journal of General Internal Medicine.* 21: 1133–7.

Carpenter, C.J. (2010) A meta-analysis of the effectiveness of Health Belief Model variables in predicting behavior. *Health Communication,* 25(8): 661–9.

Carver, C.S. and Scheier, M.F. (1998) *On the Self Regulation of Behaviour.* New York: Cambridge University Press.

Celano, C.M. and Huffman, J.C. (2011) Depression and cardiac disease: a review. *Cardiology Review.* 19(3): 130–42.

Chamberlain, C., O'Mara-Eves A., Oliver, S., Caird, J.R., Perlen, S.M., Eades, S.J. and Thomas, J. (2013) Psychosocial interventions for supporting women to stop smoking in pregnancy. *Cochrane Database of Systematic Reviews,* Issue 10. Art. No.: CD001055. DOI: 10.1002/14651858.CD001055.pub4.

Chang, A.M., Ip, W.Y. and Cheung, T.H. (2004) Patient-controlled analgesia versus conventional intramuscular injection: a cost effectiveness analysis. *Journal of Advanced Nursing.* 46(5): 531–41.

Chida, Y. and Steptoe, A. (2009) The association of anger and hostility with future CHD: a meta-analytic review of prospective evidence. *Journal of the American College of Cardiology.* 53(11): 936–46.

Churchill, R., Moore, T.H.M., Furukawa, T.A., Caldwell, D.M., Davies, P., Jones, H., Shinohara, K., Imai, H., Lewis, G. and Hunot, V. (2013) 'Third wave' cognitive and behavioural therapies versus treatment as usual for depression. *Cochrane Database of Systematic Reviews,* Issue 10. Art. No.: CD008705.

Clark, D.M. (1986) A cognitive model of panic. *Behaviour Research and Therapy.* 24: 461–70.

Clark, L.L. and Clarke, T. (2014) Realizing nursing: a multimodal biopsychopharmacosocial approach to psychiatric nursing. *Journal of Psychiatric Mental Health Nursing.* 21(6): 564–71.

Clatworthy J, Bowskill R, Parham R, Rank T, Scott J, Horne R. (2009) Understanding medication non-adherence in bipolar disorders using a Necessity-Concerns Framework. *Journal of Affective Disorders.* 116(1–2): 51–5.

Cohen, S., Gottlieb, B.H. and Underwood, L.G. (2000) Social relationships and health, in S. Cohen. L.G. Underwood and B.H. Gottlieb (eds) *Measuring and Intervening in Social Support*. New York: Oxford University Press, pp. 3–25.

Cohen-Katz, J., Wiley, S.D., Capuano, T., Baker, D.M., Kimmel, S. and Shapiro, S. (2005) The effects of mindfulness-based stress reduction on nurse stress and burnout, Part II: A quantitative and qualitative study. *Holistic Nursing Practice*. 19(1): 26–35.

Collins, M. (2006) Taking a lead on stress: rank and relationship awareness in the NHS. *Journal of Nursing Management*. 14(4): 310–17.

Conversano, C., Rotondo, A., Lensi, E., Della Vista, O., Arpone, F. and Reda, M.A. (2010) Optimism and its impact on mental and physical well-being. *Clinical Practice and Epidemiology in Mental Health*. 6: 25–9.

Cooney, G.M., Dwan, K., Greig, C.A., Lawlor, D.A., Rimer, J., Waugh, F.R., McMurdo, M. and Mead, G.E. (2013) Exercise for depression. *Cochrane Database of Systematic Reviews*: Issue 9. Art. No.: CD004366. DOI: 10.1002/14651858.CD004366.pub6.

Coulter, A., Roberts, S. and Dixon, A. (2013) Delivering better services for people with long-term conditions: building the house of care. The King's Fund. www.kingsfund.org.uk/sites/files/kf/field/field_publication_file/delivering-better-services-for-people-with-long-term-conditions.pdf (accessed 28/11/2014).

Coulthard, M., Farrell, M., Singleton, N. and Meltzer, H. (2002) Tobacco, alcohol and drug use and mental health. Office for National Statistics. www.google.co.uk/?gws_rd=ssl#q=Tobacco%2C+alcohol+and+drug+use+and+mental+health (accessed 28/08/2015).

Coventry, P.A. and Gellatly, J.L. (2008) Improving outcomes for COPD patients with mild-to-moderate anxiety and depression: a systematic review of cognitive behavioural therapy. *British Journal of Health Psychology*. 13(3): 381–400.

Cox, J.L., Holden, J.M. and Sagovsky, R. (1987) Detection of postnatal depression: development of the 10-item Edinburgh Postnatal Depression Scale. *British Journal of Psychiatry*. 150: 782–6.

Corrigan, P. (2004) How stigma interferes with mental healthcare. *American Psychologist*. 59(7): 614–25.

Cramp, F., Hewlett, S., Almeida, C., Kirwan, J.R., Choy, E.H.S., Chalder, T., Pollock, J. and Christensen, R. (2013) Non-pharmacological interventions for fatigue in rheumatoid arthritis. *Cochrane Database of Systematic Reviews*, Issue 8. Art. No.: CD008322. DOI: 10.1002/14651858.CD008322.pub2.

Crombez, G., Eccleston, C., Van Damme, S., Vlaeyen, J.W. and Karoly, P. (2012) Fear-avoidance model of chronic pain: the next generation. *Clinical Journal of Pain*. 28(6): 475–83.

Cross, W.F. and West, J.C. (2011) Examining implementer fidelity: conceptualizing and measuring adherence and competence. *Journal of Children's Services*. 6(1): 18–33.

Dalrymple, K.L., Fiornetino, L., Politi, M.C. and Posner, D. (2010) Incorporating principles from acceptance and commitment therapy into cognitive-behavioral therapy for insomnia: a case example. *Journal of Contemplative Psychotherapy*. 40: 209–17.

Darker, C.D., French, D.P., Eves, F.F. and Sniehotta, F.F. (2010) An intervention to promote walking amongst the general population based on an 'extended' theory of planned behaviour: a waiting list RCT. *Psychology & Health*. 25(1): 71–88.

D'Auria J.P., Christian, B., Henderson, Z. and Haynes, B. (2000) The company they keep: the influence of peer relationships on adjustment to cystic fibrosis during adolescence. *Journal of Pediatric Nursing*. 15: 175–82.

De Lusignan, S., Chan, T., Tejerina Arreal, M.C., Parry, G., Dent-Brown, K. and Kendrick, T. (2013) Referral for psychological therapy of people with long term conditions improves adherence to antidepressants and reduces emergency department attendance: controlled before and after study. *Behaviour Research and Therapy*. 51(7): 377–85.

de, Silva D. (2011) Helping people help themselves: a review of the evidence considering whether it is worthwhile to support self-management. Health Foundation. www.health.org. uk/publication/evidence-helping-people-help-themselves (accessed 27/08/2015).

Debney, M.T. and Fox, K.F. (2011) Rapid access cardiology – a nine year review. *Quarterly Journal of Medicine*. 105: 231–4.

Deci, E.L. and Ryan, R.M. (1985) *Intrinsic motivation and self-determination human behavior*. New York: Plenum.

DeWalt, D.A. and Hink, A. (2009) Health literacy and child health outcomes: a systematic review of the literature. *Pediatrics*. 124(Suppl 3): S265–74.

Diabetes UK (2010) Emotional and psychological support and care in diabetes: report from the emotional and psychological support working group of NHS Diabetes and Diabetes UK. www.diabetes.org.uk/Documents/reports/emotional_and_Psychological_Support_and_Care_in_Diabetes_2010.pdf (accessed 28/07/2015).

Dickens, C. and Piano M.R. (2013) Health literacy and nursing: an update. *American Journal of Nursing*. 113(6): 52–7.

Diener, E. and Suh, E. (1997) Measuring quality of life: economic, social, and subjective indicators. *Social Indicators Research*. 40(1–2): 189–216.

DiMatteo, M.R. (2004) Variations in patients' adherence to medical recommendations: a quantitative review of 50 years of research. *Medical Care*. 42(3): 200–9.

Dodge, R., Daly, A., Huyton, J. and Sanders, L. (2012) The challenge of defining wellbeing. *International Journal of Wellbeing*. 2(3): 222–35.

DH (2004) Physical activity, health improvement and prevention. At least five a week: evidence on the impact of physical activity and its relationship to health, in *Chief Medical Officer Annual Report*. London: DH.

DH (2005) *Self Care – a real choice*. London: DH.

DH (2009) *Your Health, Your Way: A Guide to Long Term Conditions and Self Care*. London: DH. http://webarchive.nationalarchives.gov.uk/20130107105354/www.dh.gov.uk/prod_con-sum_dh/groups/dh_digitalassets/documents/digitalasset/dh_097586.pdf (accessed 5/12/2014).

DH (2012) *Long Term Conditions Compendium of Information* (Third edition). London: DH. www.gov.uk/government/uploads/system/uploads/attachment_data/file/216528/dh_134486.pdf (accessed 28/11/2014).

Dorrian, J., Lamond, N., van den Heuvel, C., Pincombe, J., Rogers, A.E. and Dawason, D. (2006) A pilot study of the safety implications of Australian nurses' sleep and work hours. *Chronobiology International*. 23(6): 1149–63.

Dorrian, J., Tolley, C., Lamond, N., van den Heuvel, C., Pincombe, J., Rogers, A.E. and Drew, D. (2008) Sleep and errors in a group of Australian hospital nurses at work and during the commute. *Applied Ergonomics*. 39(5): 605–13.

Doull, M., O'Connor, A.M., Welch, V., Tugwell, P. and Wells, G.A. (2005) Peer support strategies for improving the health and well-being of individuals with chronic diseases (Protocol). *Cochrane Database of Systematic Reviews*, Issue 3. Art. No.: CD005352. DOI: 10.1002/14651858.CD005352.

Dragomir, A., Côté, R., Roy, L., Blais, L., Lalonde, L., Bérard, A. and Perreault, S. (2010) Impact of adherence to antihypertensive agents on clinical outcomes and hospitalization costs. *Medical Care*. 48(5): 418–25.

Driesen, K., Jansen, N.W., van Amelsvoort, L.G. and Kant, I. (2011) The mutual relationship between shift work and depressive complaints – a prospective cohort study. *Scandinavian Journal of Work Environment & Health*. 37(5): 402–10.

Duaso, M.J., McDermott, M.S., Mujika, A., Purssell, E. and While, A. (2014) Do doctors' smoking habits influence their smoking cessation practices? A systematic review and meta-analysis. *Addiction*. 109: 1811–23.

Dunn, D. (2005) Substance abuse among nurses – defining the issue. *AORN Journal*. 82(4): 573–82, 585–8, 592–96, quiz 599–602.

Edinger, J.D., Wohlgemuth, W.K., Radtke, R.A., Marsh, G.R. and Quillian, R.E. (2001) Cognitive behavioral therapy for treatment of chronic primary insomnia. *Journal of the American Medical Association*. 285: 1856–64.

Elwell, L., Povey, R., Grogan, S., Allen, C. and Prestwich, A. (2013) Patients' and practitioners' views on health behaviour change: a qualitative study. *Psychology and Health*. 28(6): 653–74.

Embuldeniya, G., Veinot, P., Bell. E., Bell, M., Nyhof-Young, J., Sale, J.E.M. and Britten, N. (2013) The experience and impact of chronic disease peer support interventions: a qualitative synthesis. *Patient Education and Counseling*. 92(1): 3–12. www.sciencedirect.com/science/article/pii/S0738399113000530 (accessed 1/12/15).

Engel, G.L. (1977) The need for a new medical model: a challenge for biomedicine. *Science*. 196: 129–36.

Eriksson, M. and Lindstrom, B. (2006) Antonovsky's sense of coherence scale and the relation with health: a systematic review. *Journal of Epidemiology and Community Health*. 60(5): 376–81.

Espie, C., Macmahon, K., Kelly, H-L., Broomfield, N.M., Fleming, L., Inglis, S.J., McKinstry, B., Morin, C.M., Walker, A., Wilson, P., Taylor, L., Walker, L., Paul, J. and Cassidy, J. (2005) Manualised CBT for insomnia delivered by nurse practitioners: results from studies conducted in primary care and in oncology. *Sleep Medicine*. 6(2).

Fass, R. and Achem, S.R. (2011) Non-cardiac chest pain: epidemiology, natural course and pathogenesis. *Journal of Neurogastroenterology and Motility*. 17:110–23.

Fennessy, M.M., Devon, H.A., Ryan, C., Lopez, J.J. and Zerwic, J.J. (2013) Changing illness perceptions and adherence to dual antiplatelet therapy in patients with stable coronary disease. *Journal of Cardiovascular Nursing*. 28(6): 573–83.

Feodor Nilsson, S., Andersen, P.K., Strandberg-Larsen, K. and Nybo Andersen, A.M. (2014) Risk factors for miscarriage from a prevention perspective: a nationwide follow-up study. *British Journal of Obstetrics & Gynaecology*. 121(11): 1375–84.

Ferguson, J., Bauld, L., Chesterman, J. and Judge, K. (2005) The English smoking treatment services: one-year outcomes. *Addiction*.100: 59–69.

Fidler, J.A. and West, R. (2009) Self-perceived smoking motives and their correlates in a general population sample. *Nicotine and Tobacco Research*. 11(10): 1182–8.

Fishbein, M. and Ajzen, I. (1975) *Belief, Attitude, Intention, and Behaviour: An Introduction to Theory and Research*. Reading, MA: Addison-Wesley.

Fishkind, A. (2002) Calming agitation with words, not drugs: 10 commandments for safety. *Current Psychiatry*.1(4): 32–34, 37–39. www.currentpsychiatry.com/fileadmin/cp_archive/pdf/0104/0104_Fishkind.pdf (accessed 20/8/2015).

Foster, G., Taylor, S.J.C., Eldridge, S., Ramsay, J. and Griffiths, C.J. (2007) Self-management education programmes by lay leaders for people with chronic conditions. *Cochrane Database of Systematic Reviews*, Issue 4. Art. No.: CD005108. DOI: 10.1002/14651858. CD005108.pub2.

Francis, R. (2013) *Report of the Mid Staffordshire NHS Foundation Trust Public Inquiry*. London: The Stationery Office.

Freedman, D.S., Khan, L.K., Serdula, M.K., Dietz, W.H., Srinivasan, S.R. and Berenson, G.S. (2005) The relation of childhood BMI to adult adiposity: the Bogalusa Heart Study. *Pediatrics*. 115(1): 22–7.

French, D.P., Darker, C.D., Eves, F.F. and Sniehotta, F.F. (2013) The systematic development of a brief intervention to increase walking in the general public using an 'extended' theory of planned behavior. *Journal of Physical Activity and Health*. 10(7): 940–8.

French, S.E., Lenton, R., Walter, V. and Eyles, J. (2000) An empirical evaluation of an expanded nursing stress scale. *Journal of Nursing Measurement*. 8: 161–78.

Freudenberger, H.J. (1974) Staff burn-out. *Journal of Social Issues*. 30(1): 159–85.

Furze, G., Bull, P., Lewin, R.J. and Thompson, D.R. (2003) Development of the York Angina Beliefs Questionnaire. *Journal of Health Psychology*. 8(3): 307–15.

Gallant, M.P. (2003) The influence of social support on chronic illness self-management: a review and directions for research. *Health Education and Behaviour*. 30(2): 170–95.

Garber, J., Clarke, G., Weersing, R., Beardslee, W.R., Brent, D.A., Gladstone, T.R.G., DeBar, L.L., Lynch, F.L., D'Angelo, E., Hollon, S.D., Shamseddeen, W. and Iyengar, S. (2009) Prevention of depression in at-risk adolescents: a RCT. *Journal of the American Medical Association*. 301(21): 2215–24.

Gardner, W.L. and Cacioppo, J.T. (1995) Multi-gallon blood donors: why do they give? *Transfusion*. 35: 795–8.

Gardner, B., Lally, P. and Wardel, J. (2012) Making health habitual: the psychology of 'habit-formation' and general practice. *British Journal of General Practice*. 62(605): 664–6.

Gavin, N.I., Gaynes, B.N., Lohr, K.N., Meltzer-Brody, S., et al. (2005) Perinatal depression: a systematic review of prevalence and incidence. *Obstet Gynecol*, 106: 1071–83.

Giles, E.L., Robalino, S., McColl, E., Sniehotta, F.F. and Adams, J. (2014) The effectiveness of financial incentives for health behaviour change: systematic review and meta-analysis. *PLoS One*. 9(3): e90347.

Gillespie, L. and Raftery, A.M. (2014) Nutrition in palliative and end-of-life care. *British Journal of Community Nursing*. (Suppl): S15–20.

Glombiewski, J.A., Hartwich-Tersek, J. and Rief, W. (2010) Two psychological interventions are effective in severely disabled, chronic back pain patients: a RCT. *International Journal of Behavioural Medicine*. 17(2): 97–107.

Gollwitzer, P.M. and Brandstatter, V. (1997) Implementation intentions and effective goal pursuit. *Journal of Personality and Social Psychology*. 73: 186–99.

Gollwitzer, P.M. and Sheeran, P. (2006) Implementation intentions and goal achievement: a meta-analysis of effects and processes. *Advances in Experimental Social Psychology*. 38: 69–119.

Goodwin, R.D., Faravelli, C., Rosi, S., Cosci, F., Truglia, E. de G.R. and Wittchen H.U. (2005) The epidemiology of panic disorder and agoraphobia in Europe. *European Neuropsychopharmacology*. 15(4): 435–43.

Greene, J. and Hibbard, J.H. (2012) Why does patient activation matter? An examination of the relationships between patient activation and health-related outcomes. *Journal of General Internal Medicine*. 27(5): 520–6.

Guo, S.W. and Wang, Y. (2006) The prevalence of endometriosis in women with chronic pelvic pain. *Gynecologic and Obstetric Investigation*. 62(3): 121–30.

Hagger, M.S. and Orbell, S. (2003) A meta-analytic review of the common-sense model of illness representations. *Psychology & Health*. 18(2): 141–84.

Hagger, M. (2010) Self-regulation: an important construct in health psychology research and practice (Editorial). *Health Psychology Review*. 4(2): 57–65.

Hagger, M.S., Wood, C., Stiff, C. and Chatzisarantis, N.L.D. (2010) Self-regulation and self control in exercise: the strength-energy model. *International Review of Sport and Exercise Psychology*. 3: 62–86.

Hajek, P., Stead, L.F., West, R., Jarvis, M., Hartmann-Boyce, J. and Lancaster, T. (2013) Relapse prevention interventions for smoking cessation. *Cochrane Database of Systematic Reviews*, Issue 8. Art. No.: CD003999. DOI: 10.1002/14651858.CD003999.pub4.

Hall, P.A. and Fong G.T. (2007) Temporal self-regulation theory: a model for individual health behavior. *Health Psychology Review*. 1: 6–52.

Halpern, S., Asch, D. and Volpp, K. (2012) Commitment Contracts as a way to health. *BMJ*. 344:e522.

Hamer, M., Molloy, G.J. and Stamatakis, E. (2008) Psychological distress as a risk factor for cardiovascular events: pathophysiological and behavioral mechanisms. *Journal of the American College of Cardiology*. 52(25): 2156–62.

Harrison, J.A., Mullen, P.D. and Green, L.W. (1992) A meta-analysis of studies of the health belief model with adults. *Health Education Research*. 7: 107–16.

Hawton, K. and van Heeringen, K. (2009) Suicide. *Lancet*. 373(9672): 1372–81.

Hayes, S.C. (2004) Acceptance and commitment therapy, relational frame theory, and the third wave of behavior therapy. *Behavior Therapy*. 35: 639–65.

Health and Safety Executive (2006) Managing shift work: health and safety guidance. Bootle: HSE. www.hse.gov.uk/toolbox/organisation/shiftwork.htm (accessed 1/12/15).

Helgeson, V.S., Reynolds, K.A., Tomich, P.L. (2006) A meta-analytic review of benefit finding and growth. *Journal of Consulting and Clinical Psychology*. 74(5): 797–816.

Hendershot, C.S., Witkiewitz, K., George, W.H. and Marlatt, G.A. (2011) Relapse prevention for addictive behaviors. *Substance Abuse Treatment, Prevention and Policy*. 6: 17.

Henderson, L.W. and Knight, T. (2012) Integrating the hedonic and eudaimonic perspectives to more comprehensively understand wellbeing and pathways to wellbeing. *International Journal of Wellbeing*. 2(3): 196–221.

Heslop, K. and Foley, T. (2009) Using cognitive behavioural therapy to address the psychological needs of patients with COPD. *Nursing Times*. 105: 18–19.

Hibbard, J.H. and Greene, J. (2013) What the evidence shows about patient activation: better health outcomes and care experiences; fewer data on costs. *Health Affairs*. 32(2): 207–14.

Ho, P.M., Magid, D.J., Shetterly, S.M., Olson, K.L., Maddox, T.M., Peterson, P.N., Masoudi, F.A. and Rumsfeld, J.S. (2008) Medication nonadherence is associated with a broad range of adverse outcomes in patients with coronary artery disease. *American Heart Journal*. 155(4): 772–9.

Hodnett, E.D., Fredericks, S. and Weston, J. (2010) Support during pregnancy for women at increased risk of low birthweight babies. *Cochrane Database of Systematic Reviews*, Issue 6. Art. No.: CD000198. DOI: 10.1002/14651858.CD000198.pub2.

Hodnett, E.D., Gates, S., Hofmeyr, G.J. and Sakala, C. (2013) Continuous support for women during childbirth. *Cochrane Database of Systematic Reviews*. Issue 7. Art. No.: CD003766. DOI: 10.1002/14651858.CD003766.pub5.

Hoefman, E., Boer, K.R., van Weert, H.C., Reitsma, J.B., Koster, R.W. and Bindels, P.J. (2007) Continuous event recorders did not affect anxiety or quality of life in patients with palpitations. *Journal of Clinical Epidemiology*. 60: 1060–66.

Hoffman, C.J., Ersser, S.J., Hopkinson, J.B., Nicholls, P.G., Harrington, J.E. and Thomas, P.W. (2012) Effectiveness of mindfulness-based stress reduction in mood, breast- and endocrine-related quality of life, and well-being in stage 0 to III breast cancer: a randomized, controlled trial. *Journal of Clinical Oncology*. 30(12): 1335–42.

Hoffmann, T.C., Glasziou, P.P., Boutron, I., Milne, R., Perera, R., Moher, D., Altman, D.G., Barbour, V., Macdonald, H., Johnston, M., Lamb, S.E., Dixon-Woods, M., McCulloch, P., Wyatt, J.C., Chan, A.W. and Michie, S. (2014) Better reporting of interventions: template for intervention description and replication (TIDieR) checklist and guide. *BMJ*. 348:g1687.

Hofmann, S.G., Sawyer, A.T. and Fang, A. (2010) The empirical status of the 'New Wave' of CBT. *Psychiatric Clinics of North America*. 33(3): 701–10.

Holmes, T.H. and Rahe, R.H. (1967) The Social Readjustment Rating Scale. *Journal of Psychosomatic Research*. 11(2): 213–8.

Holt-Lunstad, J., Smith, T.B. and Bradley Layton, J. (2010) Social relationships and mortality risk: a meta-analytic review. *PLoS Medicine*. 7(7): e1000316.

Hölzel, B.K., Carmody, J., Vangel, M., Congleton, C., Yerramsetti, S.M., Gard, T. and Lazar, S.W. (2011) Mindfulness practice leads to increases in regional brain gray matter density. *Psychiatry Research*. 191(1): 36–43.

Horne, R. (2006) Compliance, adherence, and concordance: implications for asthma treatment. *Chest*. 130(1 Suppl): 65S–72S.

Horne, R., Chapman, S.C.E., Parham, R., Freemantle, N., Forbes, A. and Cooper, V. (2013) Understanding patients' adherence-related beliefs about medicines prescribed for long-term conditions: a meta-analytic review of the Necessity-Concerns Framework. *PLoS ONE*. 8(12): e80633.

Horne, R. and Weinman, J. (1999) Patients' beliefs about prescribed medicines and their role in adherence to treatment in chronic physical illness. *Journal of Psychosomatic Research*. 47: 555–67.

Horne, R., Weinman, J. and Hankins, M. (1999) The Beliefs about Medicines Questionnaire: the development and evaluation of a new method for assessing the cognitive representation of medication. *Psychology and Health*. 14: 1–24.

Horne, R., Weinman, J., Barber, N., Elliott, R. and Morgan, M. (2006) Concordance, adherence and compliance in medicine taking. Report for the National Co-ordinating Centre for NHS Service Delivery and Organisation R & D. www.nets.nihr.ac.uk/__data/assets/pdf_file/0007/81394/ES-08-1412-076.pdf (accessed 27/08/2015).

Howard, L.M. and Ceci, C. (2013) Problematizing health coaching for chronic illness self-management. *Nursing inquiry*. 20(3): 223–31.

Howard, C. and Dupont, S. (2014) The COPD breathlessness manual: a RCT to test a cognitive-behavioural manual versus information booklets on health service use, mood and health status, in patients with COPD. *Primary Care Respiratory Medicine*. 24: 14076.

HSCIC (2014) Sickness absence rates in the NHS – January 2014 to March 2014. Health and Social Care Information Center. www.hscic.gov.uk/catalogue/PUB14544 (accessed 30/3/2015).

HSE (2007) Management standards for work related stress. Health and Safety Executive. www.hse.gov.uk/stress/standards/index.htm (accessed 30/3/2015).

Huffman, J. and Pollack, M. (2003) Predicting panic disorder among patients with chest pain: an analysis of the literature. *Psychosomatics*, 44(3): 222–36.

IAPT (2008) The IAPT Pathfinders: achievements and challenges. National Health Service. www.iapt.nhs.uk/silo/files/the-iapt-pathfinders-achievements-and-challenges.pdf (accessed 11/12/2014).

Ipsos Mori (2009) *Fitness to Practice: The Health of Healthcare Professionals*. London: DH. http://webarchive.nationalarchives.gov.uk/+/www.dh.gov.uk/prod_consum_dh/groups/dh_digitalassets/@dh/@en/@ps/documents/digitalasset/dh_113549.pdf (accessed 30/3/2015).

Irving, J.A., Dobkin, P.L. and Park, J. (2009) Cultivating mindfulness in healthcare professionals: a review of empirical studies of mindfulness-based stress reduction (MBSR). *Complementary Therapies in Clinical Practice*. 15(2): 61–6.

Ishii, A., Tanaka, M., Iwamae, M., Kim, C., Yamano, E. and Watanabe, Y. (2013) Fatigue sensation induced by the sounds associated with mental fatigue and its related neural activities: revealed by magnetoencephalography. *Behavioral and Brain Functions*. 9: 24.

Izumi, S., Nagae, H., Sakurai, C. and Imamura, E. (2012) Defining end-of-life care from perspectives of nursing ethics. *Nursing Ethics*. 19(5): 608–18.

Jackson, D., Firtko, A. and Edenborough, M. (2007) Personal resilience as a strategy for surviving and thriving in the face of workplace adversity: a literature review. *Journal of Advanced Nurs*ing. 60: 1–9

Johnson, L.R., Magnani, B., Chan, V. and Ferrante, F.M. (1989) Modifiers of patient-controlled analgesia efficacy: locus of control. Part I. *Pain*. 39(1): 1722.

Jones, C.J., Smith, H. and Llewellyn, C. (2014) Evaluating the effectiveness of health belief model interventions in improving adherence: a systematic review. *Health Psychology Review*. 8(3): 253–69.

Jones, M., Harvey, A., Marston, L. and O'Connell, N.E. (2013) Breathing exercises for dysfunctional breathing/hyperventilation syndrome in adults. *Cochrane Database of Systematic Reviews*, Issue 5. Art. No.: CD009041. DOI: 10.1002/14651858.CD009041.pub2.

Jonsbu, E., Dammen, T., Morekn, G. and Martinsen, E.W. (2010) Patients with noncardiac chest pain and benign palpitations referred for cardiac outpatient investigation: a 6-month follow-up. *General Hospital Psychiatry*. 32: 406–12.

Jonsbu, E., Dammen, T., Morken, G., Moum, T. and Martinsen, E.W. (2011) Short-term cognitive behavioral therapy for non-cardiac chest pain and benign palpitations: a randomized controlled trial. *Journal of Psychosomatic Research*. 70(2): 117–23.

Jordan, J.R. and Neimeyer, R.A. (2003) Does grief counseling work? *Death Studies*. 27: 765–86.

Jowsey, T., Yen, L. and Mathews, W. (2012) Time spent on health-related activities associated with chronic illness: a scoping literature review. *BMC Public Health*. 12: 1044.

Kales, H.C., Chen, P., Blow, F.C., Welsh, D.E. and Mellow, A.M. (2005) Rates of clinical depression diagnosis, functional impairment, and nursing home placement in coexisting dementia and depression. *American Journal Geriatric Psychiatry*. 13(6): 441–9.

Kaplan, H.B., Martin, S.S., Robbins, C. (1982) Application of a general theory of deviant behavior: self-derogation and adolescent drug use. *Journal of Health and Social Behavior*. 23(4): 274–94.

Katon, W.J., Lin, E., Russo, J. and Unutzer, J. (2003) Increased medical costs of a population-based sample of depressed elderly patients. *Archives of General Psychiatry*. 60: 897–903.

Kennedy, A., Bower, P., Reeves, D., Blakeman, T., Bowen, R., Chew-Graham, C., et al. (2013) Implementation of self management support for long term conditions in routine primary care settings: cluster randomised controlled trial. *BMJ*. 346: f2882.

Kerns, R.D., Rosenberg, R., Jamison, R.N., Caudill, M.A. and Haythornthwaite, J.H. (1997) Readiness to adopt a self-management approach to chronic pain: the Pain Stages of Change Questionnaire (PSOCQ). *Pain*. 72(1–2): 227–34.

Kessler, R.C. (2000) The epidemiology of pure and co-morbid generalized anxiety disorder: a review and evaluation of recent research. *Acta Psychiatrica Scandinavica*. 406 (Suppl): 7–13.

Kessler, R.C., Chiu, W.T., Demler, O., Merikangas, K.R. and Walters, E.E. (2005a) Prevalence, severity, and co-morbidity of 12-month DSM-IV disorders in the National Co-morbidity Survey Replication. *Archives of General Psychiatry*. 62: 617–27.

Kessler, R.C., Berglund, P., Demler, O., Jin, R., Merikangas, K.R. and Walters, E.E. (2005b) Lifetime prevalence and age-of-onset distributions of DSM-IV Disorders in the National Co-morbidity Survey Replication. *Archives of General Psychiatry*. 62(6): 593–602.

Kirk, S., Beatty, S., Callery, P., Gellatly, J., Milnes, L. and Pryjmachuk, S. (2013) The effectiveness of self-care support interventions for children and young people with long-term conditions: a systematic review. *Child: Care, Health and Development*. 39(3): 305–24.

Kirsch, B. and Tate, E. (2006) Developing a comprehensive understanding of the working alliance in community mental health. *Qualitative Health Research*. 16: 1054–74.

Kisely, S.R., Campbell, L.A., Yelland, M.J. and Paydar, A. (2012) Psychological interventions for symptomatic management of non-specific chest pain in patients with normal coronary anatomy. *Cochrane Database of Systematic Reviews*, Issue 6. Art. No.: CD004101. DOI: 10.1002/14651858.CD004101.pub5.

Knibbe, J.J. and Knibbe, N.E. (2012) Static load in the nursing profession, the silent killer? *Work*. 41(Suppl1): 5637–8.

Koenig, H.G., Meador, K.G., Cohen, H.J. and Blazer, D.G. (1988) Self-rated depression scales and screening for major depression in the older hospitalized patient with medical illness. *Journal of the American Geriatric Society*. 36(8): 699–706.

Kroenke, K. (2003) Patients presenting with somatic complaints: epidemiology, psychiatric co-morbidity and management. *International Journal of Methods in Psychiatric Research.* 12(1): 34–43.

Kroenke, K., Spitzer, R.L. and Williams, J.B.W. (2001) The PHQ-9: validity of a brief depression severity measure. *Journal of General Internal Medicine.* 16: 606–13.

Kroenke, K., Spitzer, R.L., Williams, J.B. and Löwe, B. (2007) Anxiety disorders in primary care: prevalence, impairment, co-morbidity, and detection. *Annals of Internal Medicine.* 146(5): 317–25.

Kübler-Ross, E. (1969) *On Death and Dying.* New York: Macmillan.

Kurtz, S., Silverman, J., Benson, J. and Draper, J. (2003) Marrying content and process in clinical method teaching: enhancing the Calgary-Cambridge guides. *Academic Medicine.* 78(8): 802–9.

Kurtz, S.M., Silverman, J.D. and Draper, J. (1998) *Teaching and Learning Communication Skills in Medicine.* Oxford: Radcliffe Medical Press.

Kwasnicka, D., Presseau, J., White, M. and Sniehotta, F.F. (2013) Does planning how to cope with anticipated barriers facilitate health-related behaviour change? A systematic review. *Health Psychology Review.* 7(2): 129–45.

Lancaster, B.M., Gadaire, D.M., Holman, K. and LeBlanc, L.A. (2015) Association between diabetes treatment adherence and parent-child agreement regarding treatment responsibilities. *Families, Systems, & Health.* 33(2): 120–5.

Lane, D., Raichand, S., Moore, D., Connock, M., Fry-Smith, A. and Fitzmaurice, D. (2013) Combined anticoagulation and antiplatelet therapy for high-risk patients with atrial fibrillation: a systematic review. *Health Technology Assessment.* 17(30): 1–188.

Lannen, P.K., Wolfe, J., Prigerson, H.G., Onelov, E. and Kreicbergs, U.C. (2008) Unresolved grief in a national sample of bereaved parents: impaired mental and physical health 4 to 9 years later. *Journal of Clinical Oncology.* 26(36): 5870–6.

Latter, S., Sibley, A., Skinner, T.C., Cradock, S., Zinken, K.M., Lussier, M.-T., Richard, C. and Roberge, D. (2010) The impact of an intervention for nurse prescribers on consultations to promote patient medicine-taking in diabetes: a mixed methods study. *International Journal of Nursing Studies.* 47: 1126–38.

Layard, R. (2005) *Happiness: Lessons from a New Science.* Penguin: London.

Lazarus, R.S. (1974) Psychological stress and coping in adaptation and illness. *International Journal of Psychiatry in Medicine.* 5: 321–33.

Lazarus, R.S. and Folkman, S. (1984) *Stress, Appraisal, and Coping.* New York: Springer.

Lengacher, C.A., Kip, K.E., Barta, M., Post-White, J., Jacobsen, P.B., Groer, M., Lehman, B., Moscoso, M.S., Kadel, R., Le, N., Loftus, L., Stevens, C.A., Malafa, M.P. and Shelton, M.M. (2012) A pilot study evaluating the effect of mindfulness-based stress reduction on psychological status, physical status, salivary cortisol, and interleukin-6 among advanced-stage cancer patients and their caregivers. *Journal of Holistic Nursing.* 30(3): 170–85.

Leventhal, H., Meyer, D. and Nerenz, D.R. (1980) The common sense representation of illness danger, in S. Rachman (ed.) *Contributions to Medical Psychology* (vol. 2). New York: Pergamon Press, pp. 7–30.

Leventhal, H., Brissette, I. and Leventhal, E.A. (2003) The common-sense model of self-regulation of health and illness, in L.D. Cameron and H. Leventhal (eds) *The Self-Regulation of Health and Illness Behaviour.* London: Routledge, pp. 42–61.

Lewin, R.J.P., Furze, G., Robinson, J., Griffith, K., Wiseman, S., Pye, M. and Boyle, R. (2002) A RCT of a self-management plan for patients with newly diagnosed angina. *British Journal of General Practice.* 52(476): 194–201.

Liddell, A., Adshead, S. and Burgess, E. (2008) *Technology in the NHS: Transforming the Patient's Experience of Care.* London: The King's Fund.

Livermore, N., Sharpe, L. and McKenzie, D. (2010) Prevention of panic attacks and panic disorder in COPD. *European Respiratory Journal*. 35: 557–63.

Lok, I.H. and Neugebauer, R. (2007) Psychological morbidity following miscarriage. *Best Practice and Research Clinical Obstetrics and Gynaecology*. 21: 229–47.

Lorig, K., Laurent, D.D., Plant, K., Krishnan, E. and Ritter, P.L. (2014) The components of action planning and their associations with behavior and health outcomes. *Chronic Illness*. 10(1): 50–9.

Lundahl, B., Moleni, T., Burke, B.L., Butters, R., Tollefson, D., Butler, C. and Rollnick, S. (2013) Motivational interviewing in medical care settings: a systematic review and meta-analysis of RCTs. *Patient Education and Counseling*. 93(2): 157–68.

Lundh, L.G. and Broman, J.E. (2000) Insomnia as an interaction between sleep interfering and sleep interpreting processes. *Journal of Psychosomatic Research*. 49: 1–12.

Lussier, J.P., Heil, S.H., Mongeon, J.A., Badger, G.J. and Higgins, S.T. (2006) A meta-analysis of voucher-based reinforcement therapy for substance use disorders. *Addiction*. 101: 192–203.

Maben, J., Peccei, R., Adams, M., Robert, G., Richardson, A., Murrels, T. and Morrow, E. (2012) Exploring the relationship between patients' experiences of care and the influence of staff motivation, affect and wellbeing. Final report. NIHR Service Delivery and Organisation programme. www.netscc.ac.uk/hsdr/files/project/SDO_FR_08-1819-213_V01.pdf (accessed 1/12/15).

Maciejewski, P.K., Zhang, B., Block, S.D. and Prigerson, H.G. (2007) An empirical examination of the stage theory of grief. *Journal of the Americal Medical Association*. 297(7): 716–23.

Maeland J.G. and Havik O.E. (1988) Self-assessment of health before and after a myocardial infarction. *Social Science and Medicine*. 27: 597–605.

Maguire, P. and Pitceathly, C. (2002) Key communication skills and how to acquire them. *BMJ*. 325: 697.

Manley, K., Hills, V. and Marriot, S. (2011) Person-centered care: Principle of Nursing Practice D. *Nursing Standard*. 31: 35–7.

Marcano Belisario, J.S., Huckvale, K., Greenfield, G., Car, J. and Gunn, L.H. (2013) Smartphone and tablet self-management apps for asthma. *Cochrane Database of Systematic Reviews*, Issue 11. Art. No: CD010013. DOI: 10.1002/14651858.CD010013.pub2.

Markland, D., Ryan, R.M., Tobin, V.J. and Rollnick, S. (2005) Motivational interviewing and self-determination theory. *Journal of Social and Clinical Psychology* 24: 811–31.

Marks, E.M., Chambers, J.B., Russell, V., Bryan, L. and Hunter, M.S. (2014) The rapid access chest pain clinic: unmet distress and disability. *Quarterly Journal of Medicine*. 107(6): 429–34.

Marlatt, A. and Gordon, J. (1985) *Relapse Prevention*. New York: Guilford Press.

Mars, T., Ellard, D., Carnes, D., Homer, K., Underwood, M. and Taylor, S.J.C. (2013) Fidelity in complex behaviour change interventions: a standardised approach to evaluate intervention integrity. *BMJ Open*.3:e003555 DOI:10.1136/bmjopen-2013-003555

Martin, D.J., Garsle, J.P. and Davis, M.K. (2000a) Relation of the therapeutic alliance with outcome and other variables: a meta-analytic review. *Journal of Consulting and Clinical Psychology*. 68: 438–50.

Martin, R., Watson, D. and Wan, C.K. (2000b) A three-factor model of trait anger: dimensions of affect, behavior, and cognition. *Journal of Personality*. 68(5): 869–97.

Maslach, C., Schaufeli, W.B. and Leiter, M.P. (2001) Job burnout. *Annual Review of Psychology*. 52: 397–422

Massey, E.K., Tielen, M., Laging, M., Beck, D.K., Khemai, R., van Gelder, T. and Weimar, W. (2013) The role of goal cognitions, illness perceptions and treatment beliefs in self-reported adherence after kidney transplantation: a cohort study. *Journal of Psychosomatic Research*. 75(3): 229–34.

May, C., Montori, V.M. and Mair, F.S. (2009) We need minimally disruptive medicine. *BMJ*. 339: b2803–603.

Mayou, R., Bryant, B., Forfar, C. and Clark, D. (1994) Non-cardiac chest pain and benign palpitations in the cardiac clinic. *British Heart Journal*. 72: 548–53.

Mayou, R., Sprigings, D. and Gilbert, T. (1999) Patients with palpitations referred for 24-hour ECG recording. *Journal of Psychosomatic Research*. 46: 491–6.

McEachan, R.R.C., Conner, M., Taylor, N.J. and Lawton, R.J. (2011) Prospective prediction of health-related behaviours with the Theory of Planned Behaviour: a meta-analysis. *Health Psychology Review*. 5(2): 97–144.

McEwen, A., West, R. and McRobbie, H. (2008) Motives for smoking and their correlates in clients attending Stop Smoking treatment services. *Nicotine and Tobacco Research*. 10: 843–50.

McGowan, L., Cooke, L.J., Gardner, B., Beeken, R.J., Croker, H. and Wardle, J. (2013) Healthy feeding habits: efficacy results from a cluster-randomized, controlled exploratory trial of a novel, habit-based intervention with parents. *American Journal of Clinical Nutrition*. 98(3): 769–77.

McIntosh, C. and Chick, J. (2004) Alcohol and the nervous system. *Journal of Neurology, Neurosurgery and Psychiatry*. 75: iii16–iii21.

McKenna, H., Slater, P., McCance, T., Bunting, B., Spiers, A. and McElwee, G. (2001) Qualified nurses' smoking prevalence: their reasons for smoking and desire to quit. *Journal of Advanced Nursing*. 35(5): 769–75.

McManus, S., Meltzer, H. and Brugha, T. (2009) Adult psychiatric morbidity in England, 2007: results of a household survey. Leeds: NHS Information Centre for Health and Social Care. www.hscic.gov.uk/pubs/psychiatricmorbidity07 (accessed 28/08/2015).

McQueen, J., Howe, T.E., Allan, L., Mains, D. and Hardy, V. (2011) Brief interventions for heavy alcohol users admitted to general hospital wards. *Cochrane Database of Systematic Reviews*, Issue 8. Art. No.: CD005191. DOI: 10.1002/14651858.CD005191.pub3.

McVicar, A. (2003) Workplace stress in nursing: a literature review. *Journal of Advance Nursing*. 44(6): 633–42.

Melzack, R. and Wall, P.D. (1982) *The Challenge of Pain*. New York: Basic Books.

Mental Health Foundation (2014) Children and Young People. www.mentalhealth.org.uk/help-information/mental-health-a-z/C/children-young-people/ (accessed 14/11/2014).

Mercer, S.W., Gunn, J., Bower, P., Wyke, S. and Guthrie, B. (2012) Managing patients with mental and physical multimorbidity. *BMJ*. 345:e5559.

Mersky, H. and Bogduk, M., and the Task Force on Taxonomy of the International Association for the Study of Pain (1994) *Classifications of Chronic Pain: Descriptions of Chronic Pain Syndromes and Definitions of Pain Terms* (Second edition). IASP: Seattle. www.iasp-pain.org/files/Content/ContentFolders/Publications2/FreeBooks/Classification-of-Chronic-Pain.pdf (accessed 12/6/2015).

Michie, S., Rumsey, N., Fussell, A., Hardeman, W., Johnston, M., Newman, S. and Yardley, L. (2008) *Improving Health: Changing Behaviour. NHS Health Trainer Handbook*. Manual: DH (Best Practice Guidance: Gateway Ref 9721).

Michie, S., Churchill, S. and West, R. (2011a) Identifying evidence-based competences required to deliver behavioural support for smoking cessation. *Annals of Behavioural Medicine*. 41: 59–70.

Michie, S., van Stralen, M. and West, R. (2011b) The behaviour change wheel: A new method for characterising and designing behaviour change interventions. *Implementation Science*. 6: 42.

Michie, S., Richardson, M., Abraham, C., Francis, J., Hardeman, W., Eccles, M.P., Cane, J. and Wood, C.E. (2013) The behavior change technique taxonomy (v1) of 93 hierarchically clustered techniques: building an international consensus for the reporting of behavior change interventions. *Annals of Behavioural Medicine*. 46(1): 81–95.

Michie, S., West, R., Campbell, R., Brown, J. and Gainforth, H. (2014) *ABC of Behaviour Change Theories: An Essential Resource for Researchers, Policy Makers and Practitioners.* www.behaviourchangetheories.com/about-book (accessed 28/08/2015).

Miller, R.W. and Rollnick, S. (1991) *Motivational Interviewing: Preparing People to Change Addictive Behaviour.* New York: Guilford Press.

Miller, R.W. and Rollnick, S. (2012a) Meeting in the middle: motivational interviewing and self-determination theory. *International Journal of Behavioral Nutrition and Physical Activity.* 9: 25.

Miller, R.W. and Rollnick, S. (2012b) *Motivational Interviewing: Helping People Change* (Third edition). London: Guildford Press.

Montgomery, P. and Dennis, J.A. (2002) Bright light therapy for sleep problems in adults aged 60+. *Cochrane Database of Systematic Reviews*, Issue 2. Art. No.: CD003403. DOI: 10.1002/14651858.CD003403.

Moore, R.K.G., Groves, D.G., Bridson, J.D., Grayson, A.D., Wong, H., Leach, A., Lewin, R.J.P. and Chester, M.R. (2007) A brief cognitive-behavioral intervention reduces hospital admissions in refractory angina patients. *Journal of Pain and Symptom Management.* 33(3): 310–16.

Moos, R.H. and Swindle, R.W. (1990) Stressful life circumstances: concepts and measures. *Stress Medicine.* 6: 171–8.

Morin, C.M., Bootzin, R.R., Buysse, D.J., Edinger, J.D., Espie, C.A. and Lichstein, K.L. (2006) Psychological and behavioral treatment of insomnia: update of the recent evidence (1998–2004). *Sleep.* 29: 1398–414

Morriss, R., Kapur, N. and Byng, R. (2013) Practice pointer: assessing risk of suicide or self harm in adults. *BMJ.* 347: f4572

Morton, R., Everard, M.L. and Elphick, H.E. (2014) Adherence in childhood asthma: the elephant in the room. *Archives of Disease in Childhood.* 99: 949–53.

Moss-Morris, R., Weinman, J., Petrie, K.J., Horne, R., Cameron, L.D. and Buick, D. (2002) The revised Illness Perception Questionnaire (IPQ-R). *Psychology and Health.* 17(1): 1–16.

Moussavi, S., Chatterji, S., Verdes, E., Tandon, A., Patel, V. and Ustun, B. (2007) Depression, chronic diseases, and decrements in health: results from the World Health Surveys. *Lancet.* 370 (9590): 851–8.

Muraven, M. and Baumeister, R.F. (2000) Self-regulation and depletion of limited resources: does self-control resemble a muscle? *Psychological Bulletin.* 126: 247–59.

Murray, C.J., Vos, T., Lozano, R., et al. (2012) Disability-adjusted life years (DALYs) for 291 diseases and injuries in 21 regions, 1990–2010: a systematic analysis for the Global Burden of Disease Study. *Lancet.* 380(9859): 2197–223.

Myrtek, M. (2001) Meta-analyses of prospective studies on CHD, type A personality, and hostility. *International Journal of Cardiology.* 79: 245–51.

National Audit of UK Pain Services (2010–2012) www.nationalpainaudit.org (accessed 12/6/2015).

National Cancer Institute (2014) *Grief, Bereavement and Coping with Loss.* www.cancer.gov/cancertopics/pdq/supportivecare/bereavement/HealthProfessional/page3 (accessed 17/10/2014).

National Centers for Health Statistics (2006) Chartbook on trends in the health of Americans 2006, special feature: pain. www.cdc.gov/nchs/data/hus/hus06.pdf (accessed 12/6/2015).

National Obesity Observatory (2011) Obesity and Mental Health: Solutions for Public Health. www.noo.org.uk/uploads/doc/vid_10266_Obesity%20and%20mental%20health_FINAL_070311_MG.pdf (accessed 25/09/2014).

Neenan, M. and Dryden, W. (2002) *Coaching: A Cognitive Behavioural Approach.* USA: Brunner-Routledge.

Neuberger, J. (2013) More care, less pathway: a review of the Liverpool Care Pathway. http://tinyurl.com/o3mbb47 (accessed 4/6/2014).

Newbury-Birch, D., Gilvarry, E., McArdle, P., Ramesh, V., Stewart, S., Walker, J., Avery, L., Beyer, F., Brown, N., Jackson, K., Lock, C.A., McGovern, R. and Kaner, E. (2009) Impact of alcohol consumption on young people: a review of reviews. www.education.gov.uk/consultations/downloadableDocs/Review%20of%20existing%20reviews%20(Full).pdf (accessed 1/12/15).

Ng, J., Thogersen-Ntoumani, E.C., Ntoumanis, N., Deci, E.L., Ryan, R., Duda, J. and Williams, G. (2012). Self-determination theory applied to health contexts: a meta-analysis. *Perspectives on Psychological Science.* 7: 325–40.

NHS (2006) The Commissioning for Quality and Innovation scheme. NHS Institute for Innovation and Improvement. www.institute.nhs.uk/commissioning/pct_portal/cquin.html (accessed 26/01/15).

NHS (2012) The NHS's role in the public's health: a report from the NHS future forum. www.gov.uk/government/uploads/system/uploads/attachment_data/file/216423/dh_132114.pdf (accessed 20/2/15).

NHS Employers (2014) NHS sickness absence rates fall further. www.nhsemployers.org/news/2014/08/sickness-absence-rates-continue-to-fall (accessed 30/3/2015).

NHS England (2014) NHS Staff Survey. www.nhsstaffsurveys.com/Caches/Files/NHS%20staff%20survey_nationalbriefing_Final%2024022015%20UNCLASSIFIED.pdf (accessed 27/3/15).

NICE (2004) CG16 Self-harm in over 8s: longer-term management. www.nice.org.uk/guidance/cg16 (accessed 14/11/2014).

NICE (2005) CG28 Depression in children and young people: identification and management. www.nice.org.uk/guidance/cg28 (accessed 1/12/15).

NICE (2007a) PH6 Behaviour change: the principles for effective interventions. www.nice.org.uk/guidance/ph6 (accessed 1/12/15).

NICE (2007b) CG53 Chronic fatigue syndrome/myalgic encephalomyelitis (or encephalopathy): diagnosis and management. www.nice.org.uk/guidance/cg53/chapter/1recommendations#/general-principles-of-care (accessed 1/12/15).

NICE (2009a) CG90 Depression in adults: recognition and management. www.nice.org.uk/guidance/cg90 (accessed 1/12/15).

NICE (2009b) CG91 Depression in adults with a chronic physical health problem: treatment and management. www.nice.org.uk/guidance/cg91 (accessed 1/12/15).

NICE (2011a) CG113 Generalised anxiety disorder and panic disorder (with or without agoraphobia) in adults: management in primary, secondary and community care. www.nice.org.uk/guidance/cg113 (accessed 1/12/15).

NICE (2011b) CG123 Common mental health problems: identification and pathways to care. www.nice.org.uk/guidance/cg123 (accessed 1/12/15).

NICE (2014a) PH49 Behaviour change: individual approaches. www.nice.org.uk/guidance/ph49 (accessed 1/12/15).

NICE (2014b) Antenatal and postnatal mental health: clinical management and service guidance. www.nice.org.uk/CG192 (accessed 1/12/15).

Nieuwlaat, R., Wilczynski, N., Navarro, T., Hobson, N., Jeffery, R., Keepanasseril, A., Agoritsas, T., Mistry, N., Iorio, A., Jack, S., Sivaramalingam, B., Iserman, E., Mustafa, R.A., Jedraszewski, D., Cotoi, C. and Haynes, R.B. (2014) Interventions for enhancing medication adherence. *Cochrane Database of Systematic Reviews*, Issue 11. Art. No.: CD000011. DOI: 10.1002/14651858.CD000011.pub4.

Nursing and Midwifery Council (2015) *The Code: Professional Standards of Practice and Behaviour for Nurses and Midwives.* London: NMC. www.nmc.org.uk/globalassets/sitedocuments/nmc-publications/revised-new-nmc-code.pdf (accessed 12/10/2015).

Nursing Standard (2015) Eat well, nurse well. http://journals.rcni.com/page/ns/campaigns/eat-well-nurse-well (accessed 1/12/15).

Nutbeam, D. (1998) Health promotion glossary. *Health Promotion International*. 13: 349–64.

Oaten, M. and Cheng, K. (2006) Longitudinal gains in self-regulation from regular physical exercise. *British Journal of Health Psychology*. 11: 717–33.

Osby, U., Brandt, L., Correia, N., Ekbom, A. and Sparen, P. (2001) Excess mortality in bipolar and unipolar disorder in Sweden. *Archives of General Psychiatry*. 58: 844–50.

Ott, C.H. (2003) The impact of complicated grief on mental and physical health at various points in the bereavement process. *Death Studies*. 27(3): 249–72.

Padesky, C. (1993) Socratic questioning: changing minds or guiding discovery? www.padesky.com/clinical-corner (accessed 1/12/15).

Padesky, C.A. and Mooney, K.A. (1990). Presenting the cognitive model to clients. *International Cognitive Therapy Newsletter*. 6: 13–14. http://padesky.com/clinical-corner/publications (accessed 15/1/16).

Pal, K., Eastwood, S.V., Michie, S., Farmer, A.J., Barnard, M.L., Peacock, R., Wood, B., Inniss, J.D. and Murray, E. (2013) Computer-based diabetes self-management interventions for adults with type 2 diabetes mellitus. *Cochrane Database of Systematic Reviews*, Issue 3. Art. No.: CD008776. DOI: 10.1002/14651858.CD008776.pub2.

Parati, G., Antonicelli, R., Guazzarotti, F., Paciaroni, E. and Mancia, G. (2001) Cardiovascular effects of an earthquake: direct evidence by ambulatory blood pressure monitoring. *Hypertension*. 38: 1093–5.

Parkash, O., Almas, A., Hameed, A. and Islam, M. (2009) Comparison of non cardiac chest pain (NCCP) and acute coronary syndrome (ACS) patients presenting to a tertiary care centre. *Journal of the Pakistan Medical Association*. 59: 667–71.

Parrott, A.C. (1999) Does cigarette smoking cause stress? *American Psychologist*. 54: 817–20.

Payne, C., Wiffen, P.J., Martin, S. (2012) Interventions for fatigue and weight loss in adults with advanced progressive illness. *Cochrane Database of Systematic Reviews*, Issue 1. Art. No.: CD008427. DOI: 10.1002/14651858.CD008427.pub2.

Perepletchikova, F. and Kazdin, A.E. (2005) Treatment integrity and therapeutic change: issues and research recommendations. *Clinical Psychology Science and Practice*. 12: 365–83.

Petersen, R., Payne, P., Albright, J., Holland, H., Cabral, R. and Curtis, K.M. (2004) Applying motivational interviewing to contraceptive counseling: ESP for clinicians. *Contraception*. 69(3): 213–17.

Petrie, K.J., Buick, D.L., Weinman, J. and Booth, R.J. (1999) Positive effects of illness reported by myocardial infarction and breast cancer patients. *Journal of Psychosomatic Research*. 47(6): 537–43.

PHE (2014) A framework for personalised care and population health for nurses, midwives, health visitors and allied health professionals. www.gov.uk/government/publications/framework-for-personalised-care-and-population-health (accessed 14/08/2015).

Phillips, L.A., Diefenbach, M.A., Kronish, I.M., Negron, R.M. and Horowitz, C.R. (2014) The necessity-concerns framework: a multidimensional theory benefits from multidimensional analysis. *Annals of Behavioural Medicine*. 48: 7–16.

Piette, J.D., Wagner, T.H., Potter, M.B. and Shillinger, D. (2004) Health insurance status, cost-related medication underuse, and outcomes among diabetes patients in three systems of care. *Medical Care*. 42: 102–9.

Pillay, T., van Zyl, H.A. and Blackbeard, D. (2014) Chronic pain perception and cultural experience. *Social and Behavioral Sciences*. 113: 151–60.

Price, A. and Hotopf, M. (2009) The treatment of depression in patients with advanced cancer undergoing palliative care. *Current Opinion in Supportive and Palliative Care*. 3: 61–6.

Price, J.R., Mitchell, E., Tidy, E. and Hunot, V. '(2008) Cognitive behaviour therapy for chronic fatigue syndrome in adults. *Cochrane Database of Systematic Reviews*, Issue 3. Art. No.: CD001027. DOI:10.1002/14651858.CD001027.pub2.

Priebe, S., Watts, J., Chase, M. and Matanov, A. (2005) Processes of disengagement and engagement in assertive outreach patients: qualitative study. *British Journal of Psychiatry*. 187: 438–43.

Prigerson, H.G., Horowitz, M.J., Jacobs, S.C., Parkes, C., Aslan, M., Goodkin, K., Raphael, B., Marwit, S.J., Worman, C., Neimeyer, R.A., Bonanno, G., Block, S.D., Kissane, D., Boelen, P., Maercher, A., Litz, B.T., Johnson, J.G., First, M.B. and Maciejewski, P.K. Prigerson, H.G., Horoqitz, M., Jacobs, S.C., et al. (2009) Prolonged grief disorder: psychometric validation of criteria proposed for DSM-V and ICD-11. *PLoS Medicine*. 6:e1000121.

Prochaska, J. and Diclemente, C. (1983) Stages and processes of self-change of smoking: toward an integrative model of change. *Journal of Consulting and Clinical Psychology*. 51: 390–5.

Prochaska, J.O., DiClemente, C.C. and Norcross, J.C. (1992) In search of how people change: applications to addictve behaviors. *American Psychologist*. 47(9): 1102–14.

Proudfoot, J., Goldberg, D., Mann, A., Everitt, B., Marks, I. and Gray, I.A. (2003) Computerised, interactive, multimedia cognitive-behavioural program for anxiety and depression in general practice. *Psychological Medicine*. 33: 217–27.

Puttonen, S., Harma, M. and Hublin, C. (2010) Shift work and cardiovascular disease: pathways from circadian stress to morbidity. *Scandinavian Journal of Work, Environment & Health*. 36(2): 96–108.

Quartana, P.J., Campbell, C.M. and Edwards R.R. (2009) Pain catastrophizing: a critical review. *Expert Review of Neurotherapy*. 9(5): 745–58.

Quigley, M. (2013) Nudging for health: on public policy and designing choice architecture. *Medical Law Review*. 21(4): 588–621.

Radloff, L.S. (1977) The CES-D Scale: a self-report depression scale for research in the general population. *Applied Psychological Measurement*. 1(3): 385–401.

Rahman, A., Reed, E., Underwood, M., Shipley, M.E. and Omar, R.Z. (2008) Factors affecting self-efficacy and pain intensity in patients with chronic musculoskeletal pain seen in a specialist rheumatology pain clinic. *Rheumatology*. 47(12): 1183–92.

Rajpura, J.R. and Nayak, R. (2014) Role of illness perceptions and medication beliefs on medication compliance of elderly hypertensive cohorts. *Journal of Pharmacy Practice*. 27(1): 19–24.

Rasmussen, J.N., Chong, A. and Alter, D.A. (2007) Relationship between adherence to evidence-based pharmacotherapy and long-term mortality after acute myocardial infarction. *Journal of the American Medical Association*. 297(2): 177–86.

Rasmussen, H.N., Scheier, M.F. and Greenhouse, J.B. (2009) Optimism and physical health: a meta-analytic review. *Annals of Behavioural Medicine*. 37(3): 239–56.

RCN (2005) *At Breaking Point? A Survey of the Wellbeing and Working Lives of Nurses in 2005*. London: RCN.

RCN (2012a) *Going Upstream: Nursing's contribution to Public Health. Prevent, Promote and Protect: The RCN's Guidance for Nurses*. London: RCN. www.rcn.org.uk/data/assets/pdf_file/0007/433699/004203.pdf (accessed 20/2/15).

RCN (2012b) *Beyond Breaking Point. A Survey Report of RCN Members on Health, Wellbeing and Stress*. London: RCN. www.rcn.org.uk/__data/assets/pdf_file/0005/541778/004448.pdf (accessed 1/12/15).

RCN (2012c) *A Shift in the Right Direction*. London: RCN. www.rcn.org.uk/__data/assets/pdf_file/0010/479431/004286.pdf (accessed 30/3/2015).

RCN (2013) *Competences: An Education and Training Competence Framework for Peripheral Venous Cannulation in Children and Young People*. London: RCN. www.rcn.org.uk/__data/assets/pdf_file/0010/78679/003003.pdf (accessed 12/10/2015).

RCN (2015) Support behaviour change. RCN online learning. www.rcn.org.uk/development/practice/cpd_online_learning/support_behaviour_change (accessed 10/3/2015).

Rethink (2013) Lethal Discrimination. www.rethink.org/media/810988/Rethink%20Mental%20Illness%20-%20Lethal%20Discrimination.pdf (accessed 27/08/2015).

Riahi, S. (2011) Role stress amongst nurses at the workplace: concept analysis. *Journal of Nursing Management*. 6: 721–31.

Rice, V.H., Hartmann-Boyce, J. and Stead, L.F. (2013) Nursing interventions for smoking cessation. *Cochrane Database of Systematic Reviews*, Issue 8. Art. No.: CD001188. DOI: 10.1002/14651858.CD001188.pub4.

Richmond, J.S., Berlin, J.S., Fishkind, A.B., Holloman, G.H., Zeller, S.L., Wilson, M.P., Rifai, M.A. and Ng, A.T. (2012) Verbal de-escalation of the agitated patient: Consensus Statement of the American Association for Emergency Psychiatry Project BETA De-escalation Workgroup West. *Journal of Emergency Medicine*. 13(1): 17–25.

Roach, S. (1992) *The Human Act of Caring: A Blueprint for the Health Profession* (Revised edition). Ottawa: Canadian Hospital Association Press.

Robertson, N., Javed, N., Samani, N.J. and Khunti, K. (2008) Psychological morbidity and illness appraisals of patients with cardiac and non-cardiac chest pain attending a rapid access chest pain clinic: a longitudinal cohort study. *Heart*. 94:e12.

Rockliff, H.E., Lightman, S., Rhidian, E., Buchanan, H., Gordon, U. and Vedhara, K. (2014) A systematic review of psychosocial factors associated with emotional adjustment in in vitro fertilization patients. *Human Reproduction Update*. 20: 4594–613.

Rogers, R.W. (1975) A protection theory of fear appeals and attitude change. *Journal of Psychology*. 91: 3–114.

Rogers, R.W. (1983) Cognitive and physiological processes in fear appeals and attitude change: a revised theory of protection motivation, in B.L. Cacioppo and L.L. Petty (eds) *Social Psychophysiology: A Source Book*. London: Guildford Press, pp. 153–176.

Rohani, C., Khanjari, S., Abedi, H.A., Oskouie, F. and Langius-Eklof, A. (2010) Health index, sense of coherence scale, brief religious coping scale and spiritual perspective scale: psychometric properties. *Journal of Advanced Nursing*. 66(12): 2796–806.

Rosenstock, I.M. (1966) Why people use health services. *Milbank Memorial Fund Quarterly*. 44: 94–124.

Roth, A.D. and Pilling, S. (2015) A competence framework for psychological interventions with people with persistent physical health conditions. University College London. www.ucl.ac.uk/pals/research/cehp/research-groups/core/competence-frameworks/Psychological_Interventions_with_People_with_Persistent_Physical_Health_Problems (accessed 14/08/2015).

Rotter, J.B. (1966) Generalised expectancies for internal versus external control of reinforcement. *Psychological Monographs*. 80(609): 1–28.

Rowlands, G. and Nutbeam, D. (2013) Health literacy and the inverse information law. *British Journal of General Practice*. 63(608): 120–1.

Royal College of Physicians, Royal College of Psychiatrists (2013) *Smoking and Mental Health*. Royal College of Physicians. www.rcplondon.ac.uk/sites/default/files/smoking_and_mental_health_-_key_recommendations.pdf (accessed 27/08/2015).

Rutledge, T. and Hogan, B.E. (2002) A quantitative review of prospective evidence linking psychological factors with hypertension development. *Psychosomatic Medicine*. 64: 758–66.

Saddichha, S. (2010) Diagnosis and treatment of chronic insomnia. *Annals of Indian Academy of Neurology*. 13(2): 94–102.

Saha, S., Chant, S. and McGrath, J. (2007) A systematic review of mortality in schizophrenia: is the differential mortality gap worsening over time? *Archives of General Psychiatry*. 64: 1123–31.

Sanders, C., Rogers, A., Gately, C. and Kennedy, A. (2008) Planning for end of life care within lay-led chronic illness self-management training: the significance of 'death awareness' and biographical context in participant accounts. *Social Science and Medicine*. 66(4): 982–93.

Sandler, R.S., Stewart, W.F., Liberman, J.N., Ricci, J.A. and Zorich, N.L. (2000) Abdominal pain, bloating, and diarrhea in the United States: prevalence and impact. *Digestive Diseases and Sciences.* 45(6): 1166–71.

Scascighini, L., Toma, V., Dober-Spielmann S. and Sprott H. (2008) Multidisciplinary treatment for chronic pain: a systematic review of interventions and outcomes. *Rheumatology.* 47(5): 670–8.

Schiøtz, M.L., Bøgelund, M., Almda, T., Jensen, B.B. and Willaing, I. (2012) Social support and self-management behaviour among patients with Type 2 diabetes. *Diabetes Medicine.* 29(5): 654–61.

Schluter, P., Turner, C., Huntington, A., Bain, C.J. and McClure, R.J. (2011) Work/life balance: the Nurses and Midwives e-cohort study. *International Nursing Review.* 58: 28–36.

Schwarzbach, M., Luppa, M., Forstmeier, S., Konig, H.-H. and Riedel-Heller, S.G. (2014) Social relations and depression in late life: a systematic review. *International Journal of Geriatric Psychiatry.* 29(1): 1–21.

Segal, Z.V., Williams, J.M.G. and Teasdale, J.D. (2001) *Mindfulness-based Cognitive Therapy for Depression: A New Approach to Preventing Relapse.* London: Guilford Press.

Sekhri, N., Feder, G.S., Junghans, C., Hemingway, H. and Timmis, A.D. (2007) How effective are rapid access chest pain clinics? Prognosis of incident angina and non-cardiac chest pain in 8762 consecutive patients. *Heart.* 93: 458–63.

Seligman, M.E.P. (2011) *Flourish – a new understanding of happiness and well-being – and how to achieve them.* London: Nicholas Brealey Publishing.

Seligman, M.E.P. and Csikszentmihalyi, M. (2000) Positive psychology: an introduction. *American Psychologist.* 55(1): 5–14.

Selye, H. (1956) *The Stress of Life.* New York: McGraw-Hill.

Service, O., Hallsworth, M., Halpern, D., Algate, F., Gallagher, R., Nguyen, S., Ruda, S., Sanders, M. with Pelenur, M., Gyani, A., Harper, H., Reinhard, J. and Kirkman, E. (2014) EAST: four simple ways to apply behavioural insights. Behavioural Insights Team. www.behaviouralinsights.co.uk/sites/default/files/BIT%20Publication%20EAST_FA_WEB.pdf (accessed 10/3/15).

Shapiro, S.L., Astin, J.A., Bishop, S.R. and Matthew, C. (2005) Mindfulness-based stress reduction for healthcare professionals: results from a randomized trial. *International Journal of Stress Management.* 12(2): 164–76.

Sharpe, J.P., Martin, N.R. and Roth, K.A. (2011) Optimism and the Big Five factors of personality: beyond neuroticism and extraversion. *Personality and Individual Differences.* 51(8): 946–51.

Sharpe, M. and Wilks, D. (2002) Fatigue. *BMJ.* 325: 480.

Shear, M.K., Simon, N., Wall, M., Zisook, S., Neimeyer, R., Duan, N., Reynolds, C., Lebowitz, B., Sung, S., Ghesquiere, A., Gorscak, B., Clayton, P., Ito, M., Nakajima, S., Konishi, T., Melhem, N., Meert, K., Schiff, M., O'Connor, M.F., First, M., Sareen, J., Bolton, J., Skritskaya, N., Mancini, A.D. and Keshaviah, A. (2011) Complicated grief and related bereavement issues for DSM-5. *Depression and Anxiety.* 28: 103–17.

Sheeran, P. (2002) Intention – behavior relations: a conceptual and empirical review. *European Review of Social Psychology.* 12(1): 1–36.

Silva, M.N., Vieira, P.N., Coutinho, S.R., Minderico, C.S., Matos, M.G., Sardinha, L.B. and Teixeira, P.J. (2010) Using self-determination theory to promote physical activity and weight control: a RCT in women. *Journal of Behavioural Medicine.* 33(2): 110–22.

Simon, G. and Ormel, J. (1995) Healthcare costs associated with depressive and anxiety disorders in primary care. *American Journal of Psychiatry.* 152(3): 352–7.

Simpson, E. and Jones, M.C. (2013) An exploration of self-efficacy and self-management in COPD patients. *British Journal of Nursing.* 22(19): 1105–9.

Smith, A., Fortune, Z., Phillips, R., Walters, P., Lee, G.A., Mann, A., Tylee, A. and Barley, E.A. (2014) UPBEAT study patients' perceptions of the effect of CHD on their lives: a cross-sectional sub-study. *International Journal of Nursing Studies*. 51(11): 1500–6.

Smith, P.J. and Blumenthal, J.A. (2013) Exercise and physical activity in the prevention and treatment of depression. *Handbook of Physical Activity and Mental Health*. London: Routledge.

Sniehotta, F.F., Schwarzer, R., Scholz, U. and Schuz, B. (2005) Action planning and coping planning for long-term lifestyle change: theory and assessment. *European Journal of Social Psychology*. 35: 565–76.

Sokol, M.C., McGuigan, K.A., Verbrugge, R.R. and Epstein, R.S. (2005) Impact of medication adherence on hospitalization risk and healthcare cost. *Medical Care*. 43(6): 521–30.

Spitzer, R.L., Kroenke, K., Williams, J.B.W. and Löwe, B. (2006) A brief measure for assessing generalized anxiety disorder: the GAD-7. *Archives of Internal Medicine*. 166: 1092–7.

Stacey, D., Légaré, F., Col, N.F., Bennett, C.L., Barry, M.J., Eden, K.B., Holmes-Rovner, M., Llewellyn-Thomas, H., Lyddiatt, A., Thomson, R., Trevena, L. and Wu, J.H.C. (2014) Decision aids for people facing health treatment or screening decisions. *Cochrane Database of Systematic Reviews*, Issue 1. Art. No.: CD001431. DOI: 10.1002/14651858.CD001431.pub4.

Stafford, L., Berk, M., Reddy, P. and Jackson, H.J. (2007) Co-morbid depression and health-related quality of life in patients with coronary artery disease. *Journal of Psychosomatic Research*. 62: 401–10.

Steinhauser, K.E., Christakis, N.A., Clipp, E.C., McNeilly, M., McIntyre, L. and Tulsky, J.A. (2000) Factors considered important at the end of life by patients, family, physicians, and other care providers. *Journal of the American Medical Association*. 284(19): 2476–82.

Stellefson, M., Dipnarine, K. and Stopka, C. (2013) The Chronic Care Model and diabetes management in US primary care settings: a systematic review. *Preventing Chronic Disease*. 10: 120180.

Steptoe, A. (ed.) (2007) *Depression and Physical Illness*. Cambridge: Cambridge University Press.

Steptoe, A. and Kivimäki, M. (2013) Stress and cardiovascular disease: an update on current knowledge. *Annual Review of Public Health*. 34: 337–54.

Steptoe, A., Deaton, A. and Stone, A.A. (2015) Subjective wellbeing, health, and ageing. *Lancet*. 385: 640–8.

St John, T., Leon, L. and McCulloch, A. (2005) *Lifetime Impacts: Childhood and Adolescent Mental Health, Understanding the Lifetime Impacts*. London: Mental Health Foundation.

Straif, K., Baan, R., Grosse, Y., Secretan, B., El Ghissassi, F.N., Bouvard, V., Altieri, A., Benbrahim-Tallaa, L. and Cogliano, V. (2007) Carcinogenicity of shift-work, painting, and fire-fighting. *Lancet Oncology*. 8(12): 1065–6.

Sullivan, L.E., Fiellin, D.A. and O'Connor, P.G. (2005) The prevalence and impact of alcohol problems in major depression: a systematic review. *American Journal of Medicine*. 118: 330–41.

Sullivan, M.J.L., Bishop, S.R. and Pivik, J. (1995) The pain catastrophizing scale: development and validation. *Psychological Assessment*. 7(4): 524–32.

Sullivan, M.J.L., Thorn, B., Rodgers, W. and Ward, C. (2004) Path model of antecedents to pain experience: experimental and clinical findings. *Clinical Journal of Pain*. 20(3): 164–73.

Sutherland, K., Leatherman, S. and Christianson, J. (2008) Paying the patient: Does it work? The Health Foundation. www.health.org.uk/publications/paying-the-patient-does-it-work/ (accessed 10/3/15).

Taylor, G., McNeill, A., Girling, A., Farley, A., Lindson-Hawley, N. and Aveyard, A. (2014) Change in mental health after smoking cessation: systematic review and meta-analysis. *BMJ*. 348: g1151.

Thaler, R. and Sunstein, C. (2008) *Nudge: Improving Decisions about Health, Wealth, and Happiness*. Connecticut: Yale University Press.

The Schizophrenia Commission (2012) *The Abandoned Illness: A Report from the Schizophrenia Commission*. London: Rethink Mental Illness.

Thomas, S.P., Groer, M., Davis, M., Droppleman, P., Mozingo, J. and Pierce, M. (2000) Anger and cancer: an analysis of the linkages. *Cancer Nursing*. 23(5): 344–9.

Thomas, V., Heath, M., Rose, D. and Flory, P. (1995) Psychological characteristics and the effectiveness of patient-controlled analgesia. *British Journal of Anaesthesia*. 74: 271–6.

Thrall, G., Lane, D., Carroll, D. and Lip, G.Y. (2006) Quality of life in patients with atrial fibrillation: a systematic review. *American Journal of Medicine*. 119(5): 448.e1–19.

Tikotzky, L. and Sadeh, A. (2010) The role of cognitive-behavioral therapy in behavioral childhood insomnia. *Sleep Medicine*. 11(7): 686–91.

Tylee, A., Barley, E.A., Hapugoda, L. and Holt, R. (2012) Physical consequences of mental illness in primary care mental health clinics, in G. Ivbijaro (ed.) *Companion to Primary Care Mental Health*. London: Radcliffe Publishing.

Utz, R.L., Caserta, M. and Lund, D. (2012) Grief, depressive symptoms, and physical health among recently bereaved spouses. *Gerontologist*. 52(4): 460–71.

Vaccarino, V., Johnson, B.D., Sheps, D.S., Reis, S.E., Kelsey, S.F., Bittner, V., Rutledge. T., Shaw, L.J., Sopko, G., Bairey Merz. C.N. and National Heart, Lung, and Blood Institute (2007) Depression, inflammation, and incident cardiovascular disease in women with suspected coronary ischemia: the National Heart, Lung, and Blood Institute-sponsored WISE study. *Journal of the American College of Cardiology*. 50: 2044–50.

van Melle, J.P., de Jonge, P., Spijkerman, T.A., Tijssen, J.G., Ormel, J., van Veldhuisen, D.J., van den Brink, R.H. and van den Berg, M.P. (2004) Prognostic association of depression following myocardial infarction with mortality and cardiovascular events: a meta-analysis. *Psychosomatic Medicine*. 66(6): 814–22.

Van't Riet, J., Sijtsema, S.J., Dagevos, H. and De Bruijn, G.-J. (2011) The importance of habits in eating behaviour: an overview and recommendations for future research. *Appetite*. 57(3): 585.

Vassilev, I., Rogers, A., Blickem, C., Brooks, H., Kapadia, D., et al. (2013) Social networks, the 'work' and work force of chronic illness self-management: a survey analysis of personal communities. *PLoS ONE*. 8(4): e59723.

Vassilev, I., Rogers, A., Sanders, C., Kennedy, A., Blickem, C., Protheroe, J., Bower, P., Kirk, S., Chew-Graham, C. and Morris, R. (2011) Social networks, social capital and chronic illness self-management: a realist review. *Chronic Illness*. 7(1): 60–86.

Verbunt, J.M., Smeets, R.J. and Wittink, H.J. (2010) Cause or effect? Deconditioning and chronic low back pain. *Pain*. 149: 428–30.

Vickers, K.S., Kircher, K.J., Smith, M.D., Petersen, L.R. and Rasmussen, N.H. (2007) Health behavior counseling in primary care: provider-reported rate and confidence. *Family Medicine*. 39(10): 730–5.

Vlaeyen, J.W.S. and Linton, S.J. (2000) Fear-avoidance and its consequences in chronic musculoskeletal pain: a state of the art. *Pain*. 85: 317–32.

Wagner, E.H. (1998) Chronic disease management: what will it take to improve care for chronic illness? *Effective Clinical Practice*. 1: 2–4.

Wakefield, J.C. (2013) DSM-5 grief scorecard: assessment and outcomes of proposals to pathologize grief. *World Psychiatry*. 12(2): 171–3.

Wallbank, S. and Hatton, S. (2011) Reducing burnout and stress: the effectiveness of clinical supervision. *Community Pratitioner*. 84: 31–5.

Walters, P., Barley, E.A., Mann, A., Phillips, R. and Tylee, A. (2014) Depression in primary care patients with CHD: baseline findings from the UPBEAT UK study. *PLoS ONE*. 9(6): e98342.

Wang, Y.C., McPherson, K., Marsh, T., Gortmaker, S.L. and Brown, M. (2011) Health and economic burden of the projected obesity trends in the USA and the UK. *Lancet*. 378: 815–25.

Waraich, P., Goldner, E.M., Somers, J.M. and Hsu, L. (2004) Prevalence and incidence studies of mood disorders: a systematic review of the literature. *Canadian Journal of Psychiatry*, 49: 124–38.

Warner, L.M., Schwarzer, R., Schüz, B., Wurm, S. and Tesch-Römer, C. (2012) Health-specific optimism mediates between objective and perceived physical functioning in older adults. *Journal of Behavioral Medicine*. 35(4): 400–6.

Warren, L. and Hunter, B. (2014) Reflecting on resilience in midwifery. *Practising Midwife*. 17(11): 21–3.

Warriner, I. (2012) Theory-based interventions for contraception: RHL commentary. The WHO Reproductive Health Library, Geneva: WHO. http://apps.who.int/rhl/fertility/contraception/cd007249_warrineri_com/en/ (accessed 10/08/2015).

Warsi, A., Wang, P.S., LaValley, M.P., Avorn, J. and Solomon, D.H. (2004) Self-management education programs in chronic disease: a systematic review and methodological critique of the literature. *Archives of Internal Medicine*. 164(15): 1641–9.

Webb, T.L. and Sheeran, P. (2006) Does changing behavioral intentions engender behavior change? A meta-analysis of the experimental evidence. *Psychological Bulletin*. 132: 249–68.

Wesselhoeft, R., Sorensen, M.J., Heiervang, E.R. and Bilenberg, N. (2013) Subthreshold depression in children and adolescents: a systematic review. *Journal of Affective Disorders*. 151(1): 7–22.

West, R. (2005) Time for a change: putting the trans-theoretical (stages of change) model to rest. *Addiction*. 100: 1036–9.

West, R., McEwen, A., Bolling, K. and Owen, L. (2001) Smoking cessation and smoking patterns in the general population: a 1 year follow-up. *Addiction*. 96: 891–902.

White, P.D., Goldsmith, K.A., Johnson, A.L., Potts, L., Walwyn, R., DeCesare, J.C., Baber, H.L., Burgess, M., Clark, L.V., Cox, D.L., Bavinton, J., Angus, B.J., Murphy, G., Murphy, M., O'Dowd, H., Wilks, D., McCrone, P., Chalder, T., Sharpe, M. and PACE trial management group (2011) Comparison of adaptive pacing therapy, cognitive behaviour therapy, graded exercise therapy, and specialist medical care for chronic fatigue syndrome (PACE): a randomised trial. *Lancet*. 377(9768): 823–36.

White, V.M., English, D.R., Coates, H., Lagerlund, M., Borland, R. and Giles, G.G. (2007) Is cancer risk associated with anger control and negative affect? Findings from a prospective cohort study. *Psychosomatic medicine*. 69(7): 667–74.

Whitmarsh, A., Koutantji, M. and Sidell, K. (2003) Illness perceptions, mood and coping in predicting attendance at cardiac rehabilitation. *British Journal of Health Psychology*. 8(Pt2): 209–21.

WHO (1997) *WHOQOL Measuring Quality of Life*. Geneva: WHO.

WHO (2010) *International Statistical Classification of Diseases and Related Health Problems (ICD-10)*. Geneva: WHO.

WHO (2015) Health Literacy and Health Behaviour. www.who.int/healthpromotion/conferences/7gchp/track2/en/ (accessed 29/01/2015).

Whooley, M.A., Avins, A.L., Miranda, J. and Browner, W.S. (1997) Case-finding instruments for depression: two questions are as good as many. *Journal of General Internal Medicine*. 12: 439–45.

Wild, S., Roglic, G., Gree, A., Sicree, R. and King, H. (2004) Global prevalence of diabetes: estimates for the year 2000 and projections for 2030. *Diabetes Care*. 27(5): 1047–53.

Wilkinson, C. and Dare, J. (2014) Shades of grey: the need for a multi-disciplinary approach to research investigating alcohol and ageing. *Journal of Public Health Research*. 3(1): 180.

Williams, M. and Penman, D. (2011) *Mindfulness: A Practical Guide to Finding Peace in a Frantic World*. London: Piatkus.

Wing, R. and Jeffrey, R. (1999) Benefits of recruiting participants with friends and increasing social support for weight loss and maintenance. *Journal of Consulting and Clinical Psychology*. 1: 132–8.

Wortz, K., Cade, A., Menard, J., Lurie, S., Lykens, K., Bae, S., Jackson, B., Su, F., Singh, K. and Coultas, D. (2012) A qualitative study of patients' goals and expectations for self-management of COPD. *Primary Care Respiratory Journal*. 21(4): 384–91.

Yassi, A. and Lockhart, K. (2013) Work-relatedness of low back pain in nursing personnel: a systematic review. *International Journal of Occupational and Environmental Health*. 19(3): 223–44.

Yesavage, J.A., Brink, T.L., Rose, T.L., et al. (1982) Development and validation of a geriatric depression screening scale: a preliminary report. *Journal of Psychiatric Research*. 17(1): 37–49.

Zametkin, A.J., Zoon, C.K., Klein, H.W. and Munson, S. (2004) Psychiatric aspects of child and adolescent obesity: a review of the past 10 years. *Journal of the American Academy of Child and Adolescent Psychiatry*. 2(4): 625–41.

Zapf, D. (2002) Emotion work and psychological well-being – a review of the literature and some conceptual considerations. *Human Resource Management Review*. 12(2): 237–68.

Zapf, D., Seifert, C., Schmutte, B. and Mertini, H. (2001) Emotion work and job stressors and their effects on burnout. *Psychology and Health*. 16(5): 527–45.

Zigmond, A.S. and Snaith, R.P. (1983) The Hospital Anxiety and Depression Scale. *Acta Psychiatrica Scandinavica*. 67: 361–70.

Zisook, S. and Shear, K. (2009) Grief and bereavement: what psychiatrists need to know. *World Psychiatry*. 8(2): 67–74.

Zweitering, P.J., Knottnerus, A., Gorgels, T. and Rinkens, P. (1996) Occurrence of arrhythmias in general practice. *Scandinavian Journal of Primary Healthcare*. 14(4): 244–50.

INDEX